Occupation-Based Practice

Fostering Performance and Participation

Occupation-Based Practice

Fostering Performance and Participation

Edited by

Mary Law, PhD, OT(c)
McMaster University
Hamilton, Ontario

Carolyn M. Baum, PhD, OTR/L, FAOTA
Washington University
St. Louis, Missouri

Sue Baptiste, MHSc, OT(c)
McMaster University
Hamilton, Ontario

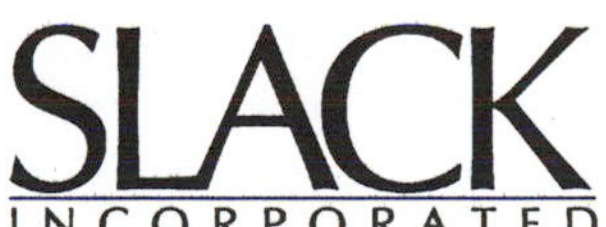

an innovative information, education, and management company

6900 Grove Road • Thorofare, NJ 08086

The procedures and practices described in this book should be implemented in a manner consistent with the professional standards set for the circumstances that apply in each specific situation. Every effort has been made to confirm the accuracy of the information presented and to correctly relate generally accepted practices. The author, editor, and publisher cannot accept responsibility for errors or exclusions or for the outcome of the application of the material presented herein. There is no expressed or implied warranty of this book or information imparted by it. Any review or mention of specific companies or products is not intended as an endorsement by the author or the publisher.

The work SLACK publishes is peer reviewed. Prior to publication, recognized leaders in the field, educators, and clinicians provide important feedback on the concepts and content that we publish. We welcome feedback on this work.

Occupation-based practice : fostering performance and participation / Mary Law, Carolyn Baum, Sue Baptiste, editors.
p ; cm.
Includes bibliographical references and index.
ISBN 1-55642-564-3 (alk. paper)
1. Occupational therapy--Practice. I. Law, Mary C. II. Baum, Carolyn Manville. III. Baptiste, Sue.
[DNLM: 1. Occupational Therapy--methods. 2. Patient-Centered Care--methods. WB 555 O1402 2001]
RM735.6 O234 2001
615.8'515--dc21

2001049593

Printed in the United States of America

Published by: SLACK Incorporated
6900 Grove Road
Thorofare, NJ 08086 USA
Telephone: 856-848-1000
Fax: 856-853-5991
www.slackbooks.com

Contact SLACK Incorporated for more information about other books in this field or about the availability of our books from distributors outside the United States.

Last digit is print number: 10 9 8 7 6 5 4 3 2 1

Contents

Acknowledgments

We wish to thank the faculty in the Department of Occupational Therapy at Washington University in St. Louis and in the School of Rehabilitation Science at McMaster University, Hamilton, Ontario, for their support and contributions to this self-study. Their commitment to this project has ensured that the practice scenarios used in the self-study reflect the diversity of occupational therapy practice. We also want to thank Lynn Snedden from McMaster University, who was instrumental in designing the layout of the self-study.

About the Editors

Mary Law, PhD, OT(c) is Professor and Associate Dean (Health Sciences), Director of the School of Rehabilitation Science, and Associate Member of the Department of Clinical Epidemiology and Biostatistics at McMaster University, Hamilton, Ontario, Canada. Mary is Co-Director of CanChild: Centre for Childhood Disability Research, a partnership between researchers at McMaster University and Children's Rehabilitation Services in Ontario. The goal of this unique partnership is to do clinically relevant research in children's rehabilitation and implement the findings into clinical practice. Mary's clinical and research interests include the development, validation, and transfer into practice of outcome measures; the study of client-centered practice; continuing validation of the Canadian Occupational Performance Measure; evaluation of therapy interventions, and the study of environmental constraints that affect the participation of children with disabilities in daily occupations.

Carolyn M. Baum, PhD, OTR/L, FAOTA is the Elias Michael Director and Associate Professor of Occupational Therapy and Neurology at Washington University School of Medicine in St. Louis, MO. Dr. Baum served as President of the American Occupational Therapy Association and President of the American Occupational Therapy Certification Board (now NBCOT). She served on the National Center for Medical Rehabilitation Research at the National Institutes of Health and the Institute of Medicine's Committee to Assess Rehabilitation Science and Engineering needs, in that capacity helping to prepare a report for Congress. Her research is on the relationship of activity and function in persons with cognitive impairment and chronic disease. She heads an interdisciplinary faculty that is contributing knowledge and training clinicians and rehabilitation scientists to understand the person and environmental factors that contribute to the performance of everyday life.

Sue Baptiste, MHSc, OT(c) is Assistant Dean of the Occupational Therapy Programme in the School of Rehabilitation Science at McMaster University. Sue came to Canada from England, pursuing an occupational therapy career that evolved into a focus on assessment and management of persons with chronic pain. Concurrently, she developed a keen interest in leadership and management, including areas of professional development, ongoing adult learning, and mentoring. Throughout her clinical and executive management career, Sue maintained a strong involvement in the academic environment and recently became a full-time faculty member at McMaster University. She has consulted around the world in areas of problem-based learning, faculty development, and curriculum reform. Her research and educational interests include the development of the Canadian Occupational Performance Measure as part of a group of six occupational therapy researchers; the development of a self-assessment tool as part of the Quality Assurance program of the College of Occupational Therapists of Ontario; and the redevelopment of the undergraduate occupational therapy curriculum.

Contributing Authors

Cynthia R. Ballentine, MSOT, OTR/L is a community practice therapist and instructor in the Program in Occupational Therapy, Washington University School of Medicine, St. Louis, MO. She currently works with the frail elderly and people with disabilities, doing assessments in order to facilitate a more supportive home environment. She also has experience in adult rehabilitation, mental health, home care, adult habilitation, long-term care, and performing driving evaluations.

Christine Berg, PhD, MS, OTR/L is an Instructor in the Program in Occupational Therapy, Washington University School of Medicine. Her areas of clinical and research interest include assessment of occupational performance in children and occupational therapy community practice in day care settings.

Mary Ann Bruce, PhD, OTR/L is Associate Director of Professional Education in the Program in Occupational Therapy, Washington University School of Medicine. Her teaching and clinical interests include psychosocial aspects of occupational performance, clinical reasoning, management and consultation, cognitive rehabilitation and adult assessment, and her research focuses on learning and problem-solving in occupational therapy education and practice.

Carol DeMatteo, MSc, OT(c) is Assistant Clinical Professor in the School of Rehabilitation Science, McMaster University. Her clinical and research interests center on occupational therapy with children with head injury and premature infants.

Kathy Kniepmann, MPH, OTR/L, CHES is an instructor and coordinator of student activities in the Program in Occupational Therapy, Washington University School of Medicine. She developed the Office of Health Education at Harvard University for students, faculty, staff, and retirees in the university community. Her professional experience includes rehabilitation, home health, and program development for health promotion, prevention, and multicultural awareness.

Patti LaVesser, PhD, OTR/L is an instructor in the Program in Occupational Therapy at Washington University. Her clinical experience is in pediatrics with emphasis in early childhood intervention, and her research interests focus on early childhood mental health and the environmental risk factors (such as prenatal drug exposure) that may contribute to child mental, behavioral, and developmental disorders.

Lori Letts, MA, OT(c) is Assistant Professor in the School of Rehabilitation Science, McMaster University. Her research centers on health promotion and ways in which community environments can support the occupational performance of older adults.

Cheryl Missiuna, PhD, OT(c) is Assistant Professor in the School of Rehabilitation Science, McMaster University. She is an investigator at CanChild: Centre for Childhood Disability Research and is doing research focused on the development and evaluation of occupational therapy interventions for children with developmental coordination disorder.

Monica S. Perlmutter, MA, OTR/L is an instructor in the Program in Occupational Therapy, Washington University School of Medicine. Her clinical experience is in adult neurology across the continuum of care. She coordinates the problem-based learning component of curriculum at Washington University.

Nancy Pollock, MSc, OT(c) is Associate Professor in the School of Rehabilitation Science, McMaster University and an investigator at CanChild: Centre for Childhood Disability Research. Her current research is focused on development of goal-setting strategies for young children and on evaluation of methods to enhance transfer of research findings into practice.

Mary Kersting Seaton, MHS, OTR/L, CHT is an Instructor in the Program in Occupational Therapy, Washington University School of Medicine. In her research, she is working on the development of the Milliken ADL Scale—a clinical instrument designed for use with persons with hand injuries—and completing work on a normative study of hand strength and its relationship to other lifestyle and anthropometric factors.

Susan Stark, PhD, OTR is an Instructor in the Program in Occupational Therapy, Washington University School of Medicine. Her clinical and research interests include the role of the environment in providing support to enhance occupational performance.

Debra Stewart, MSc, OT(c) is a clinical lecturer and professional associate in the School of Rehabilitation Science, and an associate member of CanChild: Centre for Childhood Disability Research at McMaster University.

Susan Strong, MSc, OT(c) is an Assistant Clinical Professor and research associate, Work Function Unit, School of Rehabilitation Science, McMaster University, and occupational therapist researcher at Community Schizophrenia Service, Hamilton Psychiatric Hospital, Hamilton, Ontario. Her clinical and research interests focus on issues related to participation in work and the role of environmental factors in supporting work participation.

Muriel Westmorland, MHSc, OT(c) is Associate Professor in the School of Rehabilitation Science, McMaster University. Her clinical and research interests focus on issues of transition to adulthood for youth with disabilities and transfer of research information in practice.

Laura White, BS, OT, OTR/L is a community occupational therapist in the Program in Occupational Therapy, Washington University School of Medicine. Her clinical interests include school-based practice, particularly the transition from school to work.

Seanne Wilkins, PhD, OT(c) is Assistant Professor in the School of Rehabilitation Science, McMaster University. Her research focuses on client-centered occupational therapy with older adults.

Section One

SHIFTING OUR PERSPECTIVE

When we were contemplating creating a book of this nature, the primary purpose in our minds was to ease a path through the complexities of contemporary occupational therapy practice. In our combined professional experiences, we have been part of so much professional change, from graduation when we were all prepared to perform specific tasks in response to limiting prescriptions, to the present where the roles of occupational therapists are so wide and varied that the skills required to do them well are themselves both broad and largely unfamiliar.

The practice climate has changed dramatically over the past 30 years. Currently, our societies are experiencing grand fiscal challenges, resulting in major shifts in interjurisdictional power, widely (and wildly) vacillating models for health care delivery, and an increase in conservative values, despite articulated needs for forward movement in the scope required for social service, which border on the radical.

The potential for enrichment of the occupational therapy role is massive. The loss of a traditional niche, one of comfort, should be viewed as a true opportunity for realizing important professional development and growth. There are many elements that are invitations to join the change ahead. The medical model is being challenged and physicians no longer play a global gatekeeping role, releasing the power of concepts such as health promotion and illness prevention; the emphasis on cost-effectiveness and the demand for proof of effectiveness offers a unique opportunity to illustrate the value of occupational therapy interventions; and increased interest and emphasis on complementary therapies expands the health care horizon, creating a kinder climate for new ideas.

This book is designed to be a partner for individual occupational therapists regardless of practice focus or primary role, in their exploration of developing an occupation-focused practice style based upon the complex relationships between the individuals, the environments in which they function, and the occupations with which they become involved. We, the authors, wish to welcome you, the reader, to what we believe to be an exciting and professionally fulfilling process and one essential to the continuance of a vibrant professional presence for occupational therapy.

Chapter One

Reframing Occupational Therapy Practice

Carolyn M. Baum, PhD, OTR/L, FAOTA and Sue Baptiste, MHSc, OT(c)

Goal

To foster intradisciplinary growth and collaboration around a client-centered, occupation-based practice.

Objectives of This Book

1. Enhancing knowledge to support professional identity.
2. Reaffirming and reframing skills and knowledge for occupation-based practice.
3. Facilitating transition from a focus on impairment and components to occupation and social participation.
4. Using an adult learning model to support life-long learning.

We have designed this book knowing that our occupational therapy practices are changing radically and quickly. For many years we have been centered in a medical model that by its very nature was organized around treatment and cure. Occupational therapists can take a major role in promoting health through occupation with the huge number of people who live their lives with disabilities, chronic disease, or other occupational dysfunction. Practice only within a medical model may not be the best way to achieve this goal.

This book is designed to give you ideas and tools that will help you recognize your current knowledge and place it in an occupational context. It is our goal for you to have a renewed understanding of function as occupational performance and move to a client-centered focus, no matter the specialty area of your practice.

Shifting Our Perspective

This book was created to help students and practitioners place practice in a contemporary framework. The recent *Guide to Occupational Therapy Practice* (Moyer, 1999) and *Enabling Occupation* (Canadian Association of Occupational Therapists, 1997) both support occupation-based practice as the central feature of occupational therapy. The concept of occupation is not new to occupational therapists, who have always placed value on enabling the individual to engage in activities and tasks that are meaningful and necessary. What is new is the challenge to redefine the medical model to incorporate health, wellness, and a focus on function. This redefinition requires occupational therapists to move beyond setting goals to achieve functional independence and into a client-centered approach that makes the individual's need for occupation central to the treatment process and has participation as the outcome.

Reframing Occupational Therapy Practice

Occupational therapists will continue to provide services to individuals with disabilities and chronic conditions. Perhaps what is new is that we will not just provide services in the traditional treatment environment, but we will work with individuals to reduce the risk of disablement. Services will include the individual, but will also move beyond the individual to include the family, organizations, and community agencies who provide population-based services.

As our profession changes, the field of rehabilitation is being enhanced with new knowledge in rehabilitation science. Additionally, the World Health Organization (WHO) has created an expanded model—the International Classification of Functioning (ICF) (2001), which requires rehabilitation professionals to work with consumers to implement broader models of service that explicitly address the importance of the environment as it supports or creates barriers limiting to individuals' occupational performance. This shift will place the occupational therapist in key positions within communities to foster universal design, expand the consumer's understanding of technology, and promote function and wellness in the workplace and home. Table 1-1 provides an overview of the model and integrates occupational therapy language with the International Classification of Function, Disability, and Health (2000).

The occupational therapist has always held the values that support these new roles—this book uses a series of case studies to enable the practitioner to reframe his or her current knowledge. Additionally, this book creates expanded options for occupational therapists to assume leadership roles that will ensure that their role in health and wellness, as well as in rehabilitation, will be well understood.

By going through the process in this book, you will recognize what you know already, what you need to know, and what you want to know as you reshape your approach to practice.

Over the past few years, there have been massive changes in health care systems, necessitating similar shifts in the constellation of professional roles and responsibilities for clinicians within many health care disciplines. These shifts require more sophistication in clinical reasoning, critical thinking, and therefore in the comfort level of all clinicians in accepting professional accountability for what they do, and in performing their roles in an autonomous manner.

Models of practice organized with a person-environment-occupation (PEO) focus have emerged in the last 15 years. These models are conceptually compatible with community health approaches and services that focus on health promotion and disease prevention, as well as institution-based services. These models are gaining rapid acceptance in clinical practice. The scientists and practitioners contributing to PEO models are making an important contribution to the process and also to the clients whom the profession serves.

PEO models go far beyond the issues of performance components. They, however, do not prohibit the therapist from working with the client on strategies to address performance component issues that can influence the person's occupational performance. PEO models show great promise and offer occupational therapy practitioners guidance in developing innovative and effective client-centered practice. It is not the intent of this workbook to present the individual models, but rather provide the student or practitioner with the experience of exploring how the person, environment, and occupation factors are central to planning and implementing care. The following models address the interaction of the person, his or her environment, and the activities and tasks that allow them to fulfill his or her everyday occupations:

- The Model of Human Occupation (Kielhofner & Burke, 1985; Kielhofner, 1992, 1995).
- The Person-Environment-Occupational Performance Model (Christiansen, 1991; Christiansen & Baum, 1997).
- Occupational Adaptation (Schkade & Schultz, 1992).
- The Ecology of Human Performance Model (Dunn, Brown, & McGuigan, 1994).
- Contemporary Task-Oriented Approach (Mathiowetz & Bass Haugen, 1994).
- The Person-Environment-Occupation Model (Law, Cooper, Strong, Stewart, Rigby, & Letts, 1996).
- Canadian Model of Occupational Performance (CAOT, 1997).

Inherent in the concept of professional autonomy are several assumptions that have a lasting impact on the potential success of practitioners to continue to function effectively throughout their careers. Included in these assumptions are the concepts of life-long learning, self-awareness, and self-assessment. It is upon these premises that the underlying philosophy of self-directed learning is built. This, then, is the approach we are using in this independent learning module. We are going to assist you, the learner, in developing your own learning plan, your own framework for your journey toward an occupation-based practice for the new health care reality. Think about these questions and write down your thoughts.

Table 1-1 Relating the ICF (ICIDH-2) Framework to Occupational Therapy

ICIDH Dimension	***Body Function or Structure***	***Activity/Participation***	***Environmental Factors***
PEO Terms	*Person*	*Occupation*	*Environment*
Occupational Therapy Classification	Performance components	Occupational performance	Environmental/ contextual factors
Examples of attributes	Balance Cognition (attention, planning, initiation, error detection, etc.) Endurance/strength Head control Language production Learning/memory Mood/motivation Motor planning Movement/manipulation Pain Perception Posture/sitting balance Proprioception/kinesthesis Range of motion Reflexes Sensation/touch Taste/smell Tone Vision/audition	Child care Correspondence Dressing Driving Eating Fitness Grooming Home maintenance Housekeeping Laundry Meal preparation Mobility/home, community Money management Play/leisure School Shopping Social relationships Sports Volunteer work Work Writing	Architecture/design Attitudes Cultural norms Economic policies Education Geography Health services Housing Institutions Light Family/friends Financial resources Signs Social rules Sound Surfaces Transportation Weather

➡ What changes have I experienced that have made me realize I need to look at how I will practice occupational therapy?

➡ What does life-long learning mean to me?

In order to move forward with developing an innovative approach to practice, we need to establish an ongoing process for learning, one that moves us away from the more traditional teaching methods and toward more innovative adult learning models. Although studying textbooks, attending lectures, participating in clinical skills workshops, and practicing new techniques all have a place in our life-long learning plans, there remain other opportunities to build on the ways in which adults like to learn best. This is where self-study workbooks such as this one come in.

Research into different forms of learning has identified that learning methods can be classified into three discrete categories: formal education, informal education, and non-formal education. We all engage in formal education throughout our recognized educational years, from kindergarten to perhaps as far as university; we all experience informal educational experiences continually throughout our lives from friends, family, the media, and so on. It is the non-formal educational category within which self-directed efforts can be placed, and it is constituted by having identified learners with clear objectives exploring and learning from outside the established formal system (Percy, Burton & Withnall, 1994).

➡ How do I think I learn best?

There has been a great deal of attention paid to how adults do learn best. For example, Penland (1979) established that about two-thirds of learners in his study sample preferred to study and learn in the comfort of their own home, and that the preferred method was reading from a book. Obviously, with the advent of home computers and the enhancement of computer literacy skills, this preference has likely changed; however, other findings remain relatively constant. For example, non-formal learners tend to identify that they like the flexibility to learn at their own pace, in their own time, using resources to which they are guided in part and which they identify for themselves as well (Percy et al., 1994).

➡ What will my own self-study plan look like?

- ✧ Where do I study best?
- ✧ Do I like reading from a book or the computer screen?
- ✧ What other elements have to be in place to make sure I get the most out of this opportunity?

The following chapters have been organized to act as a guide through a process of learning, as well as a process of critical thinking and critical reasoning. As you proceed through the content, there is another stream to which we would draw your attention: the development of a learning plan.

➠ Do I have a clear picture of what I want to learn from this workbook?

✧ Outline my objectives

Why Focus on Function (Occupational Performance)?

The concept of function has always been a central focus of occupational therapy and so it remains. Other professions are beginning to recognize its importance and are placing increased value on function. Fisher (1992) acknowledged that the common goal of promoting functional independence is shared by occupational therapy, physical therapy, nursing, social work, psychology, and medicine, among others. A shift is occurring throughout the health professions from a focus on pathology to a focus on function as one of the primary indicators of treatment effectiveness (Stein & Jessop, 1993). This shift also brings to the forefront the issues that occupational therapy have always valued—the person's capacity to function in a community context.

The unique term used by occupational therapy to express function is *occupational performance*. Occupational performance reflects the "individual's dynamic experience of engaging in daily occupations within the environment" (Baum & Law, 1997). The founders of occupational therapy were committed to the importance of occupation and the preservation of function (Peloquin, 1991), and early clinical efforts focused on the role of work and productivity to maintain or improve function (Hopkins, 1988). The concept of function and occupation have coexisted since the profession's inception in 1917. The following provides a short historical review of the occupational therapy profession's focus:

- 1922—Any activity, mental or physical, medically prescribed and guided for the distinct purpose of contributing to and hastening recovery from disease or injury.
- 1924—Occupational therapy aims to furnish a scheme of scientifically arranged activities which will give to any set of muscles or related parts of the body in cases of disease or injury just the degree of movement and exercise that may be directed by a competent physician or surgeon.
- 1972—The art and science of directing man's participation in selected tasks to restore, reinforce, and enhance performance; facilitate learning of those skills and functions essential for adaptation and productivity; diminish or correct pathology; and to promote and maintain health.
- 1977—Occupational therapy is the application of occupation, any activity in which one engages for evaluation, diagnosis, and treatment of problems interfering with functional performance in persons impaired by physical illness or injury, emotional disorder, congenital or developmental disability, or the aging process in order to achieve optimum function.
- 1981—Occupational therapy is the use of purposeful activity with individuals who are limited by physical injury or illness, psychosocial dysfunction, developmental or learning disabilities, poverty and cultural differences, or the aging process in order to maximize independence, prevent disability, and maintain health.
- 1990s—The definition of occupational therapy has evolved to be centered around two constructs: occupation and occupational performance. The occupational therapist employs a PEO model to help the client recover from impairments and learn new skills to carry out those activities that are personally meaningful and necessary. This model requires a client-centered approach.

"Occupation is a central aspect of the human experience and is unique to each individual; the need to engage in purposeful occupation is innate and related to health and survival" (Wilcock, 1993, p. 17). Occupation is self-directed and includes functional tasks and activities in which the person engages in over the lifespan. Occupations meet intrinsic needs for self-maintenance, expression, and fulfillment within the context of personal roles and environments (Law et al., 1996).

Occupational performance reflects the individual's dynamic experience of engaging in daily occupations (self-care, work, school, and productive pursuits) within the environment. Intervention is planned with consideration of the cultural, economic, institutional, political, and social context of the client and the family in addition to the impairment and functional limitations associated with the acute or chronic condition.

The concept of client-centered practice, which emerged from the work of Carl Rogers, has become the central concept of Canadian occupational therapy and has been adopted by clinicians and educators around the world. "Client-centered practice... embraces a philosophy of respect for, and partnership with, people receiving services. [It] recognizes the autonomy of individuals... the need for client choice... the strengths clients bring to a therapy encounter, [and] the benefits of client-therapist partnership" (Law, Baptiste, & Mills, 1995, p. 253).

➠ How do you and your colleagues define function from an occupational performance perspective?

➠ Are you comfortable using the terms *occupation* and *occupational performance* with colleagues, faculty, payers, and administrators? If not, why is using these terms difficult?

Where Does Occupational Therapy Fit into the Bigger Picture of Health?

Rehabilitation is a staged process by which physical, sensory, or mental capacities are developed or restored. This is achieved not only through behavioral changes in the person but also through changes in the physical and social environments. Rehabilitation strives to reverse what has been called the disabling process and may therefore be called the enabling process (Institute of Medicine, 1997).

Health systems define rehabilitation as a service continuum. It is traditionally thought of as acute rehabilitation, subacute care, rehabilitation, outpatient, home health, and skilled nursing. To patients, rehabilitation is a process that motivates and supports them as they learn new skills or regain their capacity to live their lives. There are four rehabilitation stages a person completes to achieve independence (McColl, Gerein, & Valentine, 1997). Some individuals move through these stages quickly, while others require a more deliberate progression through the stages. Occupational therapy services must be available to support people (and their families) at each of these stages if we are going to use our knowledge and skills to improve the occupational performance of those we serve.

Stage One: Biomedical Rehabilitation

This stage is defined as a goal-oriented and time-limited process aimed at enabling an impaired person to reach an optimum mental, physical, and/or social functional level (United Nations, 1983). In this phase of rehabilitation, a team of rehabilitation professionals collaborates to assess and diagnose the functional problems of the person. The team usually sets the goals and priorities, implements interventions to promote function, and discontinues care often according to guidelines and payment criteria (Bakheit, 1995). Biomedical rehabilitation treatment is usually focused on resuming basic self-care and developing means to support communication, movement, and performance. Specific intervention strategies are used to overcome problems, such as neglect, weakness, poor balance, and language production, among others. According to McColl and colleagues (1997), several assumptions underlie the biomedical rehabilitation stage: 1) an impairment is causing the disability, 2) problems can be analyzed into components and solved systematically, and 3) professionals have the knowledge and skill to help the patient overcome the disabling condition.

➡ What aspect of occupational therapy practice is centered in the biomedical phase of rehabilitation?

Stage Two: Client-Centered Rehabilitation

This stage shifts the focus to the person who seeks assistance of professionals to facilitate his or her problem solving and achievement of goals. Client-centered care has the capacity to help the person improve self-esteem, mastery, and resourcefulness (Emener, 1991; Goodall, 1992). Client-centered rehabilitation supports an individualized approach to therapy (Brown, 1992) and provides clients with opportunities to learn new strategies in order to perform activities that are essential to them and their families. In this phase of rehabilitation, clients identify therapeutic goals and activities that are pertinent to their unique circumstances and environments. Rehabilitation professionals support the client in learning strategies that will help him or her successfully perform activities; in other words, the practitioner presents opportunities for learning, engagement, and adaptation. This requires the health professional to move from one who takes charge and makes things better to one who facilitates change (McColl, et al., 1997).

➡ What aspect of occupational therapy practice is centered in the client-centered phase of rehabilitation?

Stage Three: Community-Based Rehabilitation

This stage is defined as a community strategy to equalize opportunities and social integration of people with disabilities (McColl et al., 1997). This means removing architectural and attitudinal barriers to foster participation in work, recreation, and family activities. This stage is implemented through the efforts of people with disabilities, their families, their communities, and professionals who see their role as an advocate. It also requires the support of health, education, vocational, social services, and the professionals who work within these systems, to work to influence policy and systems that will facilitate community participation. The assumption of community-based rehabilitation is that people with disabilities should not have their activities limited by barriers that could be removed. It also supports that individuals and communities can make a difference and by changing at a community level, the quality of life of all people in a community can improve (McColl et al., 1997).

➡ What aspect of occupational therapy practice is centered in the community-based phase of rehabilitation?

Stage Four: Independent Living

Independent living emerged from a collective political movement of persons with disabilities (DeJong, 1979; Oliver, 1990). Many people with disabilities do not want to accept dependent relationships; this includes not wanting to be dependent on a professional. They want to live their lives. The disability community developed a new approach to service delivery (independent living) to help people with disabilities access housing, health care, transportation, employment, education, and mobility.

The goal of independent living is to ensure the individual has access to resources and full participation in society (Cole, 1979). Although this goal may seem similar to traditional rehabilitation, it differs in the way the goal is addressed. The initiative for control of the service rests with the individuals themselves rather than with professionals or institutions (Cole, 1979), although the rehabilitation center can enable this process by linking with independent living centers and using peer counselors early in the rehabilitation process.

The strength of the independent living approach is its commitment to placing control in the hands of the people (DeJong, 1979). An independent living approach assumes that people with disabilities are rational and informed. It also assumes that the disability stems from the limits of the environment, not the individual (Institute of Medicine, 1997), and that disability is a lifelong personal issue, not a lifetime medical issue (McColl et al., 1997).

➡ What aspect of occupational therapy practice is centered in the independent living phase of rehabilitation?

Because occupational therapy engages with other colleagues in the rehabilitation field and many in the medical and social service communities, it is important to share a common language. The following terms should foster communication.

Additionally, in the 1990s the rehabilitation community gained consensus on its terminology. Occupational therapists need to use the following terms as they interface with professionals, administrators, and policy-makers.

Key Rehabilitation Terminology and Concepts

- Pathophysiology—The interruption or interference of normal physiological and developmental processes or structures (National Center for Medical Rehabilitation Research, 1993).
- Impairment—Loss and/or abnormality of mental, emotional, physiological, or anatomical structure or function (NCMRR, 1993).
- Functional limitation—Restriction or lack of ability to perform an action or activity in the manner or within the range considered normal that results from impairment or failure of an individual to return to the pre-existing level or function (NCMRR, 1993).
- Disability—Inability or limitation in performing socially defined activities and roles expected of individuals within a social and physical environment as a result of internal or external factors and their interplay (NCMRR, 1993).
- Environments—Those contexts that naturally occur outside the person. These contexts can facilitate or limit independence of individuals (Carver & Rodda, 1978)—as such, the environment is the context for people's performance.
- Societal Limitation—Societal policy, attitudes, and actions (or lack of), that create physical, social, or financial barriers to access health care, housing, and vocational/avocational opportunities (NCMRR, 1993).
- Handicap—A disadvantage for a given individual resulting from an impairment or a disability that limits or prevents the fulfillment of a role that is normal (depending on age, sex, and social and cultural factors) for that individual (Fougeyrollas, 1995).
- Social participation—"Nature and extent of a person's involvement in life situations" (WHO, 1998).
- Activity level—"Nature and extent of functioning at the level of the person" (WHO, 1998).

Occupational Therapy Practice: Focusing on Occupational Performance

This article was modified with permission from AOTA. Baum, C. M., & Law, M. (1997). Occupational therapy practice: Focusing on occupational performance. American Journal of Occupational Therapy, *51(4), 277-288.*

Occupational therapy practice has evolved over nearly eight decades to serve the needs of persons in a number of environments, which include health institutions, schools, work sites, and community. Until recently, practice patterns and payment mechanisms placed a greater emphasis on institutional care, where the focus of occupational therapy often addressed performance components rather than occupational performance needs of persons.

Occupational therapy is unique. Occupational therapy enables clients to achieve their goals by helping them overcome problems that limit their occupational performance. It is important to address the needs of society as it struggles with issues of chronic disease, disability, and handicapping situations. To societies, these issues mean lost productivity and costly services; to individuals they mean poorer health and a compromised well-being. About 35 million Americans, one in seven, and 4 million Canadians, 15% (Statistics Canada, 1992), have a physical or mental impairment that interferes with their daily activities, yet only 25% are so severe that they cannot work or participate in their communities. Disability is now a public health problem, affecting not only individuals with disabling conditions and their immediate families, but also society (Pope & Tarlov, 1991).

Health is viewed as much more than the absence of disease. Our health systems are being re-engineered with an emphasis on health promotion and disease prevention; building healthy communities; reducing illness, disability, and death; improving the physical environment; and ensuring accessible and affordable health services for all (Premier's Council on Health, Well-Being and Social Justice, 1993).

Over the last two decades we have seen a shift in how business is conducted and how health care is delivered. Occupational therapists and all health professionals must ensure that their services are understood by providers and clients who may not have a health knowledge base. The emergence of clinical reasoning is directly related to needing to make explicit what we know and to be understood by others. This self-study is designed to help you acquire the knowledge, confidence, and skills to make your practice of occupational therapy understood by others.

Occupational therapists need to access information to work collaboratively and to meet the needs of our clients. For example, rather than a specialist working with the sensory integrative needs of children, as occupational therapists we are now working on teams (clinical service lines), addressing the rehabilitation or habilitation needs of children, which goes far beyond the child's sensory integrative needs to include all factors that affect the child's performance.

Being effective in this new age of health care requires educated individuals who know how to work with and achieve the goals of the organization as a whole. Occupational therapists have a tradition of stepping to the forefront in times of reform when the rights of individuals are being compromised by service not directed to support the individual. We must understand the changing system to move into a position of action.

Hospitals and health care agencies are changing out of a mutual need to reach common objectives and a willingness to share risks, costs, knowledge, and capabilities. Occupational therapists recognize that many of these changes make good sense. It is not logical or cost-effective to have empty beds, to bypass large discounts for purchasing, or to have multiple hospitals staffed and equipped to do open heart or transplant surgery. There are some benefits of inter-organizational cooperation: the opportunity to learn and adapt to new competencies; to gain access to resources; to share risks, including the cost of products and technology development; to manage uncertainty; and to solve complex problems (Kaluzny, Zuckerman, & Ricketts, 1995). With this cooperation, there are some costs. Health professionals are feeling these costs, which include a loss of autonomy and control; conflict over domains, goals, and methods; and delays in solutions due to coordination problems (Kaluzny et al., 1995).

This is not the first time our profession has had to function in a changing system, although it is important to recognize that we have not had a major reform in health care in the United States since Medicare and Medicaid were initiated in the mid 1960s. As a consequence, most occupational therapists in the United States have built their professional careers in a fee-for-service system that is dissolving, and they do not have the historical perspective to see that the profession has endured many changes in the last eight decades.

A Context for Effective Occupational Therapy Practice

Occupation is a term that describes the interaction of the individual with his or her self-directed life activities. Adolph Meyer (1922), the neuroscientist, psychiatrist, and a founder of occupational therapy, proposed that "the proper use of time in some helpful and gratifying activity appears to be a fundamental issue in the [management] of any neuropsychiatric patient" (p. 1). He professed that individuals should attain and retain a healthful "rhythm in sleep and waking hours, of hunger and its gratification, and finally the big four—work and play and rest and sleep" (p. 3). Wilcock (1993) challenges us to view "occupation [as] a central aspect of the human experience and unique to each individual" (p. 17). The definition of occupation should be basic to every occupational therapist's vocabulary. Occupation meets the [individual's] intrinsic needs for self-maintenance, expression, and fulfillment within the context of personal roles and environment (Law et al., 1996). Thus, it is through the process of engagement in occupation that people develop and maintain health. Conversely, the lack of occupation causes a breakdown in habits that leads to physiological deterioration and lessens the ability to perform competently in daily life (Kielhofner, 1992). As the health system changes to focus its concern on the long-term health needs of people, issues surrounding occupation become central to promoting health and reducing the cost of chronic disability.

In her 1961 Eleanor Clark Slagle lecture, Reilly asked, "Is occupational therapy a sufficiently vital and unique service for medicine to support and society to reward?" (Reilly, 1962). Wilma West (1968) and Geraldine Finn (1972) pleaded with our profession to adopt interventions to support the health and function of persons in their communities. We no longer can ignore these challenges.

Engagement in occupation is the way that individuals maintain both cognitive and physiological fitness. Reilly (1962) tells us that "there is a reservoir of sensitivity and skill in the hands of man which can be tapped for his health [and a] rich adaptability and durability of the central nervous system which can be influenced by experience" (p. 89). As our colleagues in nursing, medicine, and physical therapy use terminology and approach their care with the intent of improving function, it is important that we make our unique contribution to function visible and understood. The term occupational therapists use for function is *occupational performance*, or the point when the person, the environment, and the person's occupation intersect to support the tasks, activities, and roles that define that person as an individual. Figure 1-1 provides a graphic representation of occupational performance.

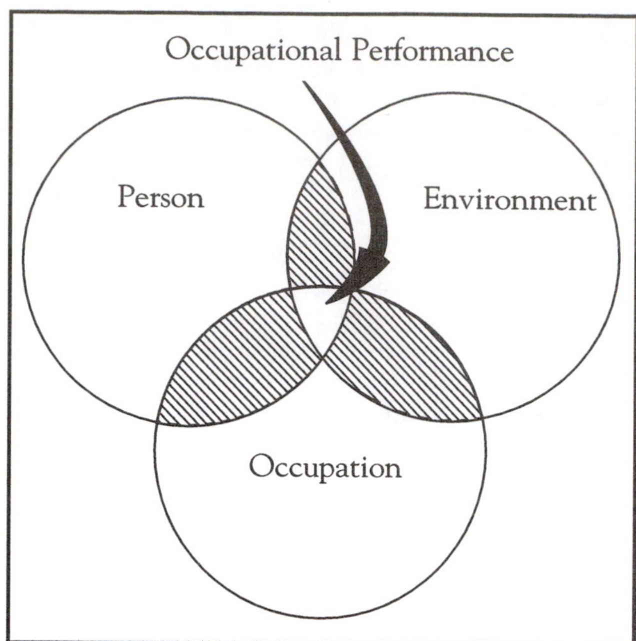

Figure 1-1. Occupational performance (reprinted with permission from the Canadian Association of Occupational Therapists, from Law, et al. (1996). The person-environment-occupation model: A transactive approach to occupational performance. *Canadian Journal of Occupational Therapy:63 (1),* 9-23).

Being able to do occupations requires the integration of factors within the individual and those external to the individual (i.e., culture, economics, resources, and the physical and social environment). Of particular interest is how these environmental factors interact with the occupational structure of the individual. Individuals who perceive that they have control over their environment and can address obstacles derive satisfaction from their occupational roles (Burke, 1977; Sharrott & Cooper-Fraps, 1986). Thus, the unique contribution of occupational therapy is to maximize the fit between what it is the individual wants and needs to do and his or her capability to do it.

The system is changing quickly and mechanisms to meet community health needs are currently being developed by our large community health systems under the label of disease management. Disease management is a comprehensive, integrated approach to care and reimbursement based on the natural course of a disease. Intervention is designed to address the illness by maximizing the effectiveness and efficiency of service delivery. Disease management differs from care paths in that it attempts to encompass the entire course of a disease, whether it is in an acute phase or remission, and whether the care is delivered in the hospital, home, or community. This process also considers the consequences of the condition across time. The purpose of these initiatives is to help people develop healthy behaviors to not only improve their health but also to cut health care costs that would be associated with dysfunction. Much of this work is currently occurring with nursing and health educators.

Occupational therapists can learn from the experiences of therapists in other countries, who have had to address similar issues. In Canada, occupational therapists were challenged by their government nearly 20 years ago to put in place a quality assurance system that would demonstrate effectiveness by improving the health of those receiving occupational therapy services (CAOT and Department of National Health and Welfare, 1983). Rather than only focus on the process of therapy, the therapists who accepted this challenge proposed a client-centered model of occupational therapy practice that spans from the institutional-based services to the community. The continuing work in Canada and developmental work in the United States can build on an emerging health system paradigm.

A community model requires occupational therapists to move beyond the medical model, which focuses on cure and management of the disease where the key relationship is between the patient and physician (Jesion & Rudin, 1983). The social (community) model focuses on the psychosocial, as well as medical, needs of individuals and encourages people to be as autonomous as possible, providing opportunities for choice in decisions and activities (Smith & Eggleston, 1989).

Occupational therapy practice has been limited by the health care system's focus on acute medical management. Recent changes in the health systems have resulted in subacute, rehabilitation, home health, and work-related programs becoming integrated parts of the system. Soon, community health initiatives, networks with independent living centers, schools, fitness and wellness programs, and vocational rehabilitation will become integral to the system. The team that historically focused on acute med-

Table 1-2 A Changing Health System Paradigm

	Old	*New*
The Model	Medical model	Sociopolitical (community model)
	Episodic care	Planned or managed health
The Focus	Focus on illness	Focus on wellness
	Acute care outcomes satisfaction	Well-being, function, and life
	Individual	Individual within the environment
	Deficiency	Capability
	Survival	Functional ability/quality of life
	Professionally controlled	Personal responsibility flexible/choice
	Dependence	Interdependence/participation
	Treatment	Treatment/prevention
The System	Institution centered	Community centered
	Single facility	Networked system
	Competitive focus	Collaborative focus
	Fragmented service	Coordinated service

ical care has been limited primarily to traditional medical rehabilitation professionals, including physicians, occupational therapists, physical therapists, speech language pathologists, psychologists, and rehabilitation nurses. The community approach expands rehabilitation to include a whole new cadre of colleagues, including people with disabilities, engineers, architects, personal assistants, independent living counselors, recreation and exercise personnel, city planners, law enforcement, and transportation specialists. See Table 1-2 for a summary of these changes.

Occupational therapists should be seen as experts in applying effective intervention strategies that contribute to optimal occupational function, including self-sufficiency, social integration, improved health status, and employment in persons with chronic disease and disability. They must work in partnerships to develop strategies to manage health problems and prevent secondary disabling conditions that can compromise function and translate directly into increased medical costs. Although many of the changes associated with this shift are painful, the ultimate goal which puts more focus on prevention fits well with the philosophy and tenets of occupational therapy with its focus on supporting the healthful behaviors and function of individuals in their daily lives.

Occupational therapists must assume the responsibility to shape their own future in the changing system. Basic to implementing a model to manage the long-term health and occupational needs of an individual is placing value on the individual directing his or her own care. Occupational therapists' terminology and programs are described as patient-centered, client-centered, patient-focused, client-driven, partnerships, family-centered—what does this mean and how do we ensure that we are leaders in shifting the paradigm?

There are some key concepts that must be mastered to describe how occupational therapy fits into a larger context of medicine and rehabilitation. The traditional approach to medical care has focused on impairments or the loss and/or abnormality of mental, emotional, physiological, or anatomical structure or function; this includes all losses or abnormalities, not just those attributable to the initial pathophysiology, and also includes pain as a limiting experience. When there is an interruption or interference of normal physiological and developmental processes or structures, the term that is used is *pathophysiology* (NCMRR, 1993).

Acute rehabilitation usually focuses on functional limitations, which are restrictions or lack of ability to perform an action or activity in the manner or within the range considered normal, that result from impairment or failure of an individual to return to the pre-existing level or function (NCMRR, 1993). This is synonymous with occupational therapists' description of performance components. In contrast, disability is defined as the inability or limitation in performing socially defined activities and roles expected of individuals within a social and physical environment as a result of internal or external factors and their interplay (NCMRR, 1993).

As the occupational therapist approaches problem solving with clients, three sets of information must be considered in planning treatment. Person factors that must be considered are neurobehavioral, cognitive, physical, and psychosocial strengths and deficits presented by the person. Environmental factors include the cultural, economic, institutional, political, and social context from the perspective of the person. Occupational factors include the self-maintenance, work, home, leisure, and family roles and activities of the person. We will look at these factors as we work through future chapters.

Now that we have begun on this journey of reframing our practice, the first stop along the way is to explore the central concept of partnership. If we are to subscribe to the key changes illustrated in the health care systems of today, then we will see the importance of the consumer movement in the development of increased awareness and involvement in decisions concerning personal health and well-being. This leads us on to Chapter Two.

References

Bakheit, A. M. O. (1995). Delivery of rehabilitation services: An integrated hospital-community approach. *Clinical Rehabilitation*, 9, 142-149.

Baum, C. M., & Law, M. (1997). Occupational therapy practice: Focusing on occupational performance. *Am J Occup Ther*, *51*(4), 277-288.

Brown, S. J. (1992). Tailoring nursing care to the individual client: Empirical challenge of a theoretical concept. *Res Nurs Health*, *15*, 39-46.

Burke, J. P. (1977). A clinical perspective on motivation: Pawn versus origin. *Am J Occup Ther*, *31*(4), 254-258.

Canadian Association of Occupational Therapists. (1997). *Enabling occupation: An occupational therapy perspective*. Ottawa, ON: CAOT Publications ACE.

Canadian Association of Occupational Therapists & Department of National Health and Welfare. (1983). *Guidelines for the client-centered practice of occupational therapy* (H39-33/1983E). Ottawa, ON: Department of National Health and Welfare.

Carver, V., & Rodda, M. (1978). *Disability and the environment*. London: Elek Books.

Christiansen, C., & Baum, C. M. (Eds.) (1991). Occupational therapy: Intervention for life performance. In C. Christiansen & C. M. Baum (Eds.), *Occupational therapy: Overcoming human performance deficits*. Thorofare, NJ: SLACK Incorporated, 4-43.

Christiansen, C., & Baum, C. M. (Eds.) (1997). *Occupational therapy: Enabling function and well-being* (2nd ed.). Thorofare, NJ: SLACK Incorporated.

Cole, J. A. (1979). What's new about independent living. *Archives of Physical Medicine and Rehabilitation*, *60*, 458-461.

DeJong, G. (1979). Independent living: From social movement to analytic paradigm. *Archives of Physical Medicine and Rehabilitation*, *60*, 435-446.

Dunn, W., Brown, C., & McGuigan, A. (1994). Ecology of human performance: A framework for considering the effect of context. *Am J Occup Ther*, *48*(7), 595-607.

Emener, W. G. (1991). Empowerment in rehabilitation: An empowerment philosophy for rehabilitation in the 20th century. *Journal of Rehabilitation*, *57*(4), 7-12.

Finn, G. L. (1972). The occupational therapist in prevention programs, 1971 Eleanor Clarke Slagle Lecture. *Am J Occup Ther*, *26*, 59-66.

Fisher, A. G. (1992). The Foundation-Functional measures, Part 1: What is function, what should we measure, and how should we measure it? *Am J Occup Ther*, *46*, 183-185.

Fougeyrollas, P. (1995). Documenting environmental factors for preventing the handicap creation process. *Disabil Rehabil*, *17*, 145-153.

Goodall, C. (1992). Preserving dignity for disabled people. *Nursing Standard*, 6(35), 25-27.

Hopkins, H. L. (1988). An historical perspective on occupational therapy. In H. L. Hopkins & H. D. Smith (Eds.), *Willard and Spackman's Occupational Therapy* (7th ed.) (pp. 16-37). Philadelphia: J.B. Lippincott Company.

International Classification of Function, Disability, and Health (2000). Revision Meeting. Madrid: World Health Organization.

Institute of Medicine. (1997). *Enabling America: Assessing the role of rehabilitation science and engineering*. E. N. Brandt Jr. & A. M. Pope (Eds.) Washington, D.C.: National Academy Press.

Jesion, M., & Rudin, S. (1983). Evaluation of the social model of long term care. *Health Management Forum, Summer*, 64-80.

Kaluzny, A. D., Zuckerman, H. S., & Ricketts, T. C. (Eds.). (1995). *Partners for the dance: Forming strategic alliances in health care*. Ann Arbor, MI: Health Administration Press.

Kielhofner, G. (1992). *Conceptual foundations of occupational therapy*. Philadelphia: F. A. Davis.

Kielhofner, G. (1995). *A model of human occupation: Theory and application* (2nd ed.). Baltimore: Williams & Wilkins.

Kielhofner, G., & Burke, J. (1985). *A model of human occupation: Theory and application*. Baltimore: Williams & Wilkins.

Law, M., Baptiste, S., & Mills, J. (1995). Client-centered practice: What does it mean and does it make a difference? *Canadian Journal of Occupational Therapy*, *62*(5), 250-257.

Law, M., Cooper, B., Strong, S., Stewart, D., Rigby, P., & Letts, L. (1996). The person-environment-occupation model: A transactive approach to occupational performance. *Canadian Journal of Occupational Therapy*, *63*(1), 9-23.

Mathiowetz, V., & Bass Haugen, J. (1994). Motor behavior research: Implications for therapeutic approaches to central nervous system dysfunction. *Am J of Occup Ther, 48*(8), 733-745.

McColl, M. A., Gerein, N., & Valentine, F. (1997). Meeting the challenges of disability: Models for enabling function and well-being. In C. Christiansen & C. Baum (Eds.), *Occupational therapy: Enabling function and well-being* (2nd ed.). Thorofare, NJ: SLACK Incorporated.

Meyer, A. (1922). The philosophy of occupation therapy. *Archives of Occupational Therapy, 1*(1), 1-10.

Moyer, P. A. (1999). The guide to occupational therapy practice. *Am J Occup Ther, 53*(3), 247-297.

National Center for Medical Rehabilitation Research. (1993). *Research plan for the National Center for Medical Rehabilitation Research*. Bethesda, MD: National Institutes of Health Publication No. 93-3509.

Oliver, M. (1990). *The politics of disablement*. London: MacMillan.

Peloquin, S. M. (1991). Occupational therapy service: Individual and collective understanding of the founders, part 1. *Am J Occup Ther, 45*(4), 352-360.

Penland, P. (1979). Self-initiated learning. *Adult Education Quarterly*, 29, 170-179.

Percy, K., Burton, D, Withnall, A. (1994). Self-directed learning among adults: the challenge for continuing educators. Leeds: Association for Lifelong Learning.

Pope, A. M., & Tarlov, A. R. (Eds.). (1991). *Disability in America: Toward a national agenda for prevention*. Washington, DC: National Academy Press.

Premier's Council on Health, Well-Being and Social Justice. (1993). *Our environment, our health*. Toronto: Province of Ontario.

Reilly, M. (1962). Occupational therapy can be one of the great ideas of 20th century medicine. *Am J Occup Ther, 16*, 87-105.

Schkade, J. K., & Schultz, S. (1992). Occupational adaptation: Toward a holistic approach to contemporary practice, Part I. *Am J Occup Ther, 46*, 829-837.

Sharrott, G. W., & Cooper-Fraps, C. (1986). Theories of motivation in occupational therapy: An overview. *Am J Occup Ther, 40*, 249-257.

Smith, V., & Eggleston, R. (1989). Long-term care: The medical versus the social model. *Public Welfare, Summer*, 26-29.

Statistics Canada. (1992). *Canadian Health and Activity Limitation Survey*. Ottawa, ON: Author.

Stein, R. E. K. & Jessop, D. J. (1993). Long-term mental health effects of a pediatric home care program. Measures for a new era of health assessment. In A. L. Stewart, & J. E. Ware. (Eds.), *Measuring functioning and well-being*. Durham: Duke University Press.

United Nations. (1983). *World program of action concerning disabled persons*. New York: United Nations.

West, W. L. (1968). Professional responsibility in times of change, 1967 Eleanor Clarke Slagle Lecture. *Am J Occup Ther, 22*, 9-15.

Wilcock, A. (1993). A theory of the human need for occupation. *Occupational Science: Australia, 1*(1), 17-24.

World Health Organization. (2001). *International Classification of Functioning—ICIDH2. Revised*. Geneva: Author.

Notes

Chapter Two

Working in Partnership with Our Clients

Mary Law, PhD, OT(c) and Sue Baptiste, MHSc, OT(c)

In Chapter Two, we will focus on the concepts underpinning client-centered practice and help you to explore ways in which these ideas influence practice. The central question we want you to think about is what does client-centered practice mean for you as an occupational therapist? When you practice from a client-centered perspective, what are the implications for you, for your client, and for the systems in which you work?

As part of exploring these ideas, we will discuss the process of learning from the client's perspective. If you think about it, learning is a constant process within the client-therapist relationship. We each begin by learning about the person's occupational performance issues, followed by factors that influence performance. We then use these to learn what makes a difference to enable the person to engage in the occupations that he or she needs or wants to do. We will describe how we have approached client learning in the past, how this has changed, and suggest learning strategies to help operationalize a true partnership between client(s) and therapists.

Let's begin by looking at client-centered practice.

Client-Centered Practice

For the past 20 years, occupational therapists have been studying, developing, and using a client-centered approach to therapy practice (Canadian Association of Occupational Therapy, 1997). Led by occupational therapists from Canada, this approach has become increasingly prominent across the world. It is fair to conclude that occupational therapy practice today is based on concepts of client-centeredness. Why does this approach to practice make sense to us? There are two primary reasons. First, a client-centered practice resonates with the fundamental values and beliefs of occupational therapy about a person's right and need to make choices, to engage in satisfying occupations, and to be supported if illness, disability, or social circumstances interfere with this. Second, a client-centered occupational therapy practice is effective. Such a practice is more likely to engage clients in the occupational therapy process and lead to increased adherence and satisfaction with therapy (Law, Baptiste, & Mills, 1995). "The goal of the [client-] centered philosophy is to create a caring, dignified, and empowering environment in which [clients] truly direct the course of their care and call upon their inner resources to speed the healing process" (Matheis-Kraft, George, Olinger, & York, 1990, p. 128).

Client-centered occupational therapy has been defined as "an approach to [service] which embraces a philosophy of respect for, and partnership with, people receiving services" (Law et al., 1995, p. 253). In a client-centered approach, clients and therapists work in partnership—each party is an expert in parts of the therapeutic process. For example, clients are the expert in identifying occupational performance issues that need occupational therapy intervention, while therapists are expert at identifying the reasons for performance difficulties in these identified tasks. Clients and therapists work together to define the focus and need for intervention, intervention strategies, and the preferred outcomes of therapy. Law (1998) has outlined the basic concepts underpinning a client-centered approach to occupational therapy practice. She has reviewed the predominant frameworks of client-centered practice and summarized the concepts that are used to describe the characteristics of this approach. These concepts include (Law, 1998, p. 9):

- Respect for clients and their families, and the choices they make.
- Clients and families have the ultimate responsibility for decisions about daily occupations and occupational therapy services.
- Provision of information, physical comfort, and emotional support with an emphasis on person-centered communication.
- Facilitation of client participation in all aspects of occupational therapy service.
- Flexible, individualized occupational therapy service delivery.
- Enabling clients to solve occupational performance issues.
- Focus on the person-environment-occupation relationship.

Let's look at how these ideas are reflected in practice. Think about what you will do or have done as an occupational therapist. Write down situations or occurrences that illustrate each of the concepts of client-centered practice listed in Table 2-1. If you cannot think of an example, spend some time reflecting on how these ideas could be made part of your future practice.

Using these assumptions that underlie client-centered practice, clients and therapists can focus on their unique contribution and responsibilities to building a client-centered partnership. In such a partnership, clients expect to fully participate in the decision-making process about occupational performance needs and desired outcomes. To do this, clients require information that will enable them to make decisions about the services that will most effectively meet their needs. This information, when given in an understandable way, will ensure that clients can define occupational performance priorities for intervention. Clients expect to receive a service in a timely manner, and to be treated with respect and dignity during occupational therapy. The therapist encourages clients to use their own resources to help solve occupational performance problems. Clients will participate at different levels, depending on their capabilities, but all are capable of making at least some choices about how they spend their daily lives.

A client-centered approach encourages occupational therapists to assume new responsibilities. Therapists will encourage client decision-making in partnership with other team members. They will also work in partnership with clients to enable them to identify their needs and individualize service provision. Client decisions are supported, or the reason why the therapist cannot support the decision is communicated to the client. There is a fundamental respect for client values and visions and for their style of coping without judging what is right and what is wrong. Clients are encouraged to recognize and build on their strengths, using natural community supports as much as possible.

What does client-centered practice not mean? A client-centered approach does not mean that therapists abrogate decision-making or that clients have the right to receive any service they believe is worthwhile. Therapists have the responsibility, both ethically and legally, to identify situations in which clients are at risk and assist them in examining such issues (CAOT, 1997). There are also issues related to fiscal resources that will have an impact on the nature and amount of occupational therapy services available.

A therapist's personal values and beliefs have an important influence on practice. It has been shown through research that beliefs and values influence the ease with which therapists engage in client-centered practice (Toomey, Nicholson, & Carswell, 1995). It is important for you to spend the time and effort to know what you believe about practicing occupational therapy. Do you support a client-centered approach to practice? What parts of this approach are difficult for you, or are not supported by the system in which you work? Know yourself well enough to know your limits so that you can say—"Yes, I agree with doing that" or "No, I don't agree with that, and here's why." With an increasingly complex and privatized health system, therapists are often faced with ethical decisions to practice in a way that does not support a client-centered practice. It is difficult to stay true to a client-centered philosophy of practice.

Think about these ideas. What are your beliefs about client-centered practice? Write them below.

➡ My beliefs about client-centered occupational therapy are:

Table 2-1 Client-Centered Practice

Concept	*Write Example(s) of How This Concept Is or Will Be Reflected in My Practice*
Respect for clients and their families, and the choices they make	
Clients and families have the ultimate responsibility for decisions about daily occupations and occupational therapy services	
Provision of information, physical comfort, and emotional support with an emphasis on person-centered communication	
Facilitation of client participation in all aspects of occupational therapy service	
Flexible, individualized occupational therapy service delivery	
Enabling clients to solve occupational performance issues	
Focus on the person-environment-occupation relationship	

➠ These aspects of practice support my beliefs:

➠ These aspects of practice are not congruent with my beliefs:

Process of Learning From a Client's Perspective

With the shift to client-centered practice, the notion of patient education takes a very different turn. If the "patient" becomes a "client," then he or she moves from a position of passive acceptance of input and information to a more active stance of involvement, engagement, and the assuming of a mantle of life-long learning. Not only is the therapist invested in continuing to learn, but he or she shares that investment with the client. Hence, one can term this innovation as facilitating client learning, rather than providing information to educate the client at one specific point in time.

Elements of adult learning can be applied to this emerging role, whether the client in question is an individual, a family or community network, an industry, private business, or government agency. In order for this role shift to be successful, the occupational therapist must begin to see herself or himself as a facilitator, a positive influence in supporting the client to assume more autonomy and responsibility for personal learning. The development of patient education materials, for example, does not have to end; rather, the task can assume a collegial edge, involving clients in creating materials and other tools which they perceive have helped them to take charge of their lives after illness or trauma.

A key approach then, to help therapists assume this new role (of facilitator of learning instead of teacher), is to develop abilities to self-assess and reflect on their own learning as a means to understand what clients experience when trying to become more independent and responsible for their on-going learning and coping. Much potentially valuable learning is lost because individuals have not taken time to reflect on how they learn best, how they retain information best, and how they operationalize what they learn (Boud, Keogh, & Walker, 1985). Clients and therapists should work toward establishing relationships that support this type of constructive reflection—developing methods of monitoring learning behaviors and the application of strategies for moving forward and gaining an increased sense of self-actualization.

Therefore, the process of self-examination through which you, the reader of this chapter, will travel can be applied equally with our clients in their quest for mastery and regained control of abilities and skills.

Planning and Implementing Client-Centered Occupational Therapy Services

An occupational therapist brings knowledge and experience to the therapeutic relationship, as does the client. When a new therapeutic relationship is evolving, it is important for the context of that relationship to be understood by both parties. It is just as important for the client to understand why an occupational therapist is involved in his or her care and what he or she can expect to achieve through occupational therapy, as it is for the therapist to understand the issues and needs of the client.

It is important for the client to understand the scope of the therapist's knowledge and access to resources. Likewise, the client's knowledge of his or her condition and experience with the problem and his or her goals must become clear for the relationship to progress. If the person has a cognitive deficit or is a child who as yet does not have the capacity for independent decision-making, the parent or the person selected to be the guardian or caretaker must participate in this phase of planning. If the occupational therapist does not have the knowledge to address the client's needs, the therapist should help the client seek the resources he or she needs to be sure that the problems presented by the client can be addressed.

In many situations, it may be easier to say that you will practice from a client-centered perspective than it is to actually do that. There are many clinical situations in which there may not be agreement or may be some conflict between the client's goals, family's goals, and health professionals or health system involved in his or her care. The challenge the occupational therapist faces in these situations is to examine these issues openly and in collaboration with the client and his or her family.

Let's look at some specific examples in which the implementation of client-centered principles into practice is challenging. We have provided a key question for you to consider when determining strategies for the implementation of client-centered practice in this particular situation. We have left room for you to add your ideas about how these situations might be approached.

Clinical Examples

Mr. Johnson is an 82-year-old man recently hospitalized because of medical frailty and difficulty looking after his basic needs. Both he and his family want him to return home to live on his own. However, assessments completed by the team, including the occupational therapist, indicate concerns regarding his safety and ability to function at home.

➠ How do you work with Mr. Johnson and his family to address this conflict?

A therapist has a client who recently moved here from Asia, a 67-year-old woman, Liu Chan, recovering from surgery to replace her hip. She has three children, all married, but living very close by. She is used to running her own household and is very involved with her family. They are prepared to help her when she tells them what she would like them to do. She is silent when talking with her therapist, since she is waiting to hear what the instructions are for her rehabilitation. She sees the therapist as the expert and would not think of saying what was bothering her or voicing her key concerns.

➠ How do you involve the client and her family in a client-centered manner?

You are a recent graduate working as an occupational therapist in a hand injury clinic. The physician and other members of the team are most interested in you collecting information and focusing on the client's range of motion, strength, and manual dexterity. Your education emphasizes the importance of focusing on the person's occupational history. The pace of work in the clinic is very fast. Your concern is that if you focus on occupational history, you'll not have as much time to collect the information that others consider very important.

➠ How can you address the occupational history concerns of the clients while still paying attention to the important component aspects of their injury?

Franz is a 50-year-old man who recently arrived from Austria. He was transferred with his multinational company—he is a senior manager in the electronics industry. Stoic, resolute, and determined to present a capable and "in-charge" demeanor, he always reports that his back pain and migraines are under control, despite evidence of increasing medication intake and additional down-time.

➠ How can you encourage this client to engage at a "real" level with his therapist in order to begin to improve his pain-coping strategies by setting realistic goals in a client-centered and occupation-based way?

Recently, you worked with a woman who had a mild stroke. She returned home and you provided home occupational therapy services to her. She stated that one of her goals was to be able to continue her leisure interest of ballroom dancing. You knew that it was unlikely that this activity goal would be approved for reimbursement.

- How can you address this very real "occupational" need of the client?

Anna is a 27-year-old woman from Colombia who escaped from her country under threat of re-imprisonment following torture and the loss of her 2-year-old child (he was taken from her, and she does not know his fate). She is working with her therapist in order to become acclimatized to her life in a new country. She is seldom forthcoming with much information and tends to remain apart, yet looks eager for input. She is tentative and does not respond easily to requests to identify areas upon which she would like to concentrate her efforts.

- How can you enable Anna to focus on an intervention plan in which she is invested while recognizing her obvious need for support and time to heal?

John, 58 years old, is a native Canadian from the Ojibwa nation. He has diabetes and has been followed by a clinic for some time. However, he is not regular in his attendances at appointments and has announced that he is going to attend a healing circle instead of coming to the diabetic day clinic as prescribed by the doctor on the reserve where he lives.

- How could his therapist be the most client-centered and occupation-based with John?

There are many factors that influence our ability as occupational therapists to practice in a client-centered manner. Supports for client-centered practice include leadership from the organization, support for continuing education, a welcoming physical environment, and continued emphasis on open and facilitative communication. Important barriers to client-centered practice that have been identified include lack of management support for this approach to service and lack of time and resources to ensure a client-centered philosophy is built into every aspect of service delivery (Law, 1998).

- Spend a few minutes thinking about your own practice or clinical situations you have visited. Identify the supports and barriers to a client-centered practice that exist right now. It helps to identify these factors in terms of yourself as a therapist, the clients you work with, and the system in which you will work.
  - Therapist
  - Clients
  - System

Planning Occupational Therapy Intervention

During the next chapters of this self-study, we will be focusing on the occupational therapy intervention process and issues that affect our ability to implement an occupation-based practice. But let's start by taking the time to look at what you do or what you are learning right now.

Think of potential clients that you will work with in your occupational therapy practice. With these people (or groups or organizations) in mind, answer the questions listed below.

- What do you do the first time you see a client?

- What do you hope to get out of the first session with a client?

- How do you approach assessment—What do you use? What do you assess first?

- How do you decide therapy goals?

- What guides you in determining what you and the client do during treatment sessions?

- How do you evaluate if your treatment makes a difference?

Now that you've thought about client-centered practice ideas and the process of your practice, let's look at your practice using a different lens. Figure 2-1 represents a way of illustrating the occupational therapy practice process as it exists in most places today.

Thinking about this process and the concepts of client-centered practice, answer the following questions:

- When you first see a client, how could you obtain his or her occupational history?

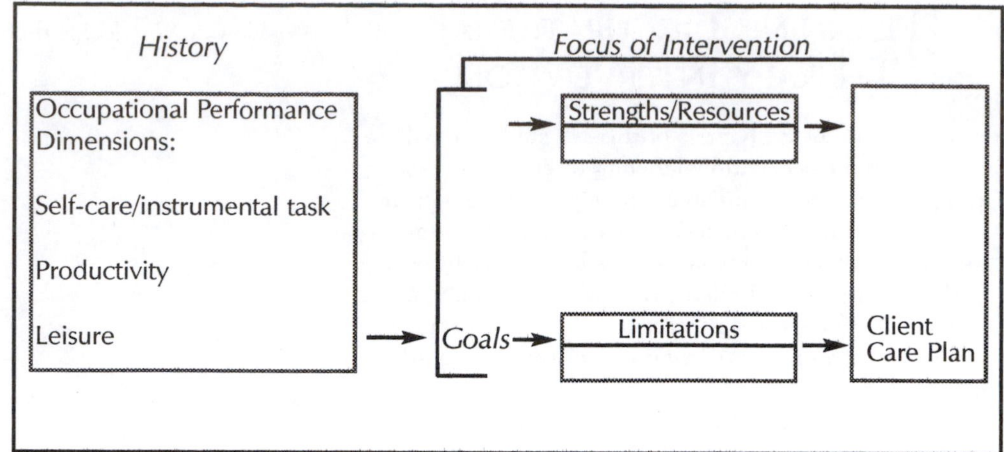

Figure 2-1. Process for care plan development.

- Do your clients identify the goals of therapy? How is this done? When is it difficult to do?

- How do you identify resources of the client, the therapists, and the environment?

- How do you identify limitations to moving forward from the client, therapist, and environment?

- Do you frame your intervention process as occupation-based? In what way(s)?

- How do you state your intervention plan and report on progress—tasks, activities, function, or occupation?

- What are the indicators of success—are they related to changes in occupational performance?

➡ How do you frame continuing goals and intervention plans?

In Chapter Two, you have learned about the concepts of client-centered occupational therapy and reflected on implementation of these ideas in your own practice. You have also read about learning from the client's perspective and how this influences your day-to-day practice. We have examined the key elements required of us in order to reorganize how we perform our practice roles in occupational therapy, and we are ready to move on into how to make it happen within the practice context. It is one thing to understand the theoretical implications and value of adopting this approach, but it is another to begin to utilize it within a work context that has been used to seeing you do your job in a certain way and, therefore, relating to you in an established manner. So, let's explore "fostering occupational performance and participation" in Chapter Three.

References

Boud, D., Keogh, R., & Walker, D. (1985). *Reflection: Turning experience into learning*. New York: Nichols Publishing Company.

Canadian Association of Occupational Therapists. (1997). *Enabling occupation: An occupational therapy perspective*. Ottawa, ON: CAOT Publications ACE.

Law, M. (Ed.). (1998). *Client-centered occupational Therapy*. Thorofare, NJ: SLACK Incorporated.

Law, M., Baptiste, S., & Mills, J. (1995). Client-centered practice: What does it mean and does it make a difference? *Canadian Journal of Occupational Therapy, 62*, 250-257.

Matheis-Kraft, C., George, S., Olinger, M. J., & York, L. (1990). Patient-driven healthcare works. *Nursing Management, 21*, 124-128.

Toomey, M., Nicholson, D., & Carswell, A. (1995). The clinical utility of the Canadian Occupational Performance Measure. *Canadian Journal of Occupational Therapy, 62*, 242-249.

Resources

Canadian Association of Occupational Therapists. (1997). *Enabling occupation: An occupational therapy perspective*. Ottawa, ON: CAOT Publications ACE.

Christensen, C., & Baum, C. (Eds.). (1997). *Occupational therapy: Enabling function and well-being* (2nd ed.). Thorofare, NJ: SLACK Incorporated.

Law, M. (Ed.). (1998). *Client-centered occupational therapy*. Thorofare, NJ: SLACK Incorporated.

Notes

Chapter Three

Fostering Occupational Performance and Participation

Carolyn M. Baum, PhD, OTR/L, FAOTA

Practice Scenario Authors:

Christine Berg, PhD, MS, OTR/L
Mary Kersting Seaton, MHS, OTR/L, CHT
Laura White, BS, OT, OTR/L

Practicing from an occupational performance perspective requires us to expand our process of clinical reasoning and expand our approach to focus on the client's needs and goals as the central aspect of treatment planning. Impairment approaches have been used in the past to conceptualize treatment that was organized to fit into a medical model. Unfortunately, an impairment-oriented approach may have unnecessarily narrowed the focus of occupational therapy to the management of impairments (performance components) and encouraged therapists to make assumptions that reducing the impairment would result in increased function. In some cases this might be true, but this approach does not meet the criteria for being client-centered or even being considered rehabilitation unless the way in which that impairment impacts everyday life is concurrently addressed. Working from a client-centered community orientation allows us to see how our practice and others' understanding of our practice has been limited by treatment focused purely in medically oriented settings. A case in point:

Mr. and Mrs. Jones

Case modified and used with permission from Law, M. (1998). Client-centered occupational therapy. *Thorofare, NJ: SLACK Incorporated.*

Mrs. Jones has diabetes. She was hospitalized and received acute occupational therapy and physical therapy services; after discharge she had home health services. She was taught basic self-care and transfer techniques; she also received a bath bench, an extended showerhead, a wheelchair, and a walker. Attention was focused on ensuring that she had the range of motion and skills to carry out her basic needs. Unfortunately, little attention was directed toward her functioning at home, particularly her loss of vision.

Mr. Jones is frail with a heart condition and needs skills to feel competent in his role as care provider. He reports that he and his wife are very isolated and that his wife has become so dependent that he is required to perform even very simple personal tasks for her. He expresses worry that he may not be able to keep up the pace required to care for her much longer.

Mr. Jones must be seen not only as the environmental support of Mrs. Jones, but also as a client whose health may be compromised by the frustrations and tasks of his role. The biomechanical and rehabilitative approaches used with Mrs. Jones focused on her impairment and basic self-care function, not Mr. and Mrs. Jones as vulnerable older adults struggling to continue to live in their own home.

The Jones' needs go far beyond what a traditional approach supports. A client-centered and occupational performance-based approach is needed. Such approaches will help them understand their options and how to integrate fitness, socialization, and meaningful occupations into their daily routines. The couple needs help that is available from community agencies like chore service and assistance with shopping and transportation. The extended family also needs skills to develop competencies to help with some of the couple's needs.

There are a number of environmental strategies that can enhance the occupational performance of both Mrs. and Mr. Jones. The lighting in the home is too dim, and she needs some visual adaptations so she can read. Mr. Jones requires new strategies for transfers until Mrs. Jones gets stronger. Mrs. Jones also needs some of her clothes adapted so that she can dress more easily. Recently she has remained in her robe all day and does not want neighbors to see her like that. Some additional assessments could help. The occupational therapist can make a difference in people's lives when the approach considers the needs and goals of the client(s).

This chapter will focus on two practice situations. We will ask you to respond to a series of questions that will help you focus your planning on occupational performance. Such an approach can make explicit the unique contribution of occupational therapy in health care whether you work in a hospital, rehabilitation facility, school, an industry, or in a community agency. First is an introduction to Alice Wilson.

Meet Alice Wilson

Alice is a 28-year-old woman who lives on a farm in a rural area with her husband and three young children, ages 4 years, 2 years, and 9 months. Her husband makes his living by farming. Alice is employed in a local manufacturing plant. Alice got her left hand caught between two rollers at work. She was able to push the emergency cut-off switch; however, her hand was caught up to the mid-metacarpal level and someone had to get her out. She was immediately taken to the emergency room. She had a crush injury without fracture, tendon, or nerve injury. A dorsal fasciotomy was performed to relieve the edema and pressure in her hand. The occupational therapist provided an intrinsic-plus position resting hand splint. Alice has now been referred for outpatient occupational therapy.

As background, we need to know that Alice carries a major role in the family. Her parents and two married sisters live in a suburban area 160 miles away (a 3-hour drive). The client and her husband moved to this rural area, where her husband grew up, to take over his father's farm when his parents retired to Florida. They know some neighbors and people at church. Alice lives in a two-story farmhouse where she is responsible for management of her home and family. Her husband takes care of the children while she works the evening shift (3 p.m. to 11 p.m.) in a local manufacturing plant to supplement the family income.

When Alice arrives for her outpatient visit, the occupational therapist administers a battery of tests that are traditional for a hand practice. These include active range of motion, passive range of motion, upper extremity edema/volume, upper extremity sensation, and the Milliken Activities of Daily Living scale. Because the occupational therapist had just returned from a class at the university, which focused on client-centered care, she also focused on asking Alice to describe her issues related to everyday functioning.

Alice's concerns:

1. Alice said her hand injury was interfering with her ability to care for her children's physical needs.
2. She needs to clean her home and cook.
3. She is worried that the hand injury is compromising the family income.
4. Though she was embarrassed to say it, she was concerned about the appearance of her hand.

Begin to make a list of Alice's strengths and limitations. If some of the information you need is not available, be sure to identify what additional issues need to be addressed.

Alice's Strengths

- Person
  - No nerve damage, no fractures

- Environmental
  - Modern home with conveniences

- Occupational
  - ✧ Write down your thoughts here

Alice's Limitations

- Person
  - ✧ Pain, uncomfortable with appearance, fear of weakness, and deconditioning
- Environmental
  - ✧ Family expectations cannot be met, family help is several hours away
- Occupational
  - ✧ Routine activities are difficult
- Her resources
  - ✧ Husband, neighbors, church members, health insurance worker's compensation

The Occupational Therapy Plan

The occupational therapy plan focuses on resolution of component and environmental issues that contribute to the client's problems:

- Problem 1: Decreased active and passive digital range of motion due to trauma with resultant edema and stiffness.
  - ✧ Approach: Implement edema reduction via elevation, compression sleeves, and active motion. Implement dynamic digital splinting with the client to apply orthosis four to six times per day for 15 to 30 minutes to a point of stretch, not pain, and follow it with active grasp and release/functional use to enhance effectiveness of the splint.
  - ✧ What could Alice do to increase motion and reduce edema when performing tasks from her everyday life demands?
- Problem 2: Appearance of hand 2 degree to trauma.
  - ✧ Approach: Resolution will be enhanced by activities to decrease edema and improve functional motion. Patient should be encouraged to discuss areas of concern and think through what could help her to feel better.
  - ✧ What activities could you introduce to help her begin to accept her hand as a useful tool?
- Problem 3: Decreased upper extremity sensation.
  - ✧ Approach: Implement a sensory re-education program to promote relearning of sensory input and to increase functional use, coupled with writing in a "use diary."

- ✧ What could Alice do to increase her sensation using tasks that her everyday life demands? (Perhaps things she could do with her children.)

- Problem 4: Role and responsibilities issues.
  - ✧ Approach: Issues of concern regarding home and work should be discussed and prioritized. Implement instruction and practice of one-handed techniques. Work out strategies for home organization with the client's husband and children. Explore support resources in the church and local community.
  - ✧ What could Alice do in therapy and at home to accomplish the tasks that support her life demands?

- Problem 5: Worksite issues.
  - ✧ Approach: Discuss concerns regarding job performance and practice simulation of targeted job task components.
  - ✧ List ideas that would facilitate Alice's return to work.

Additional problems that are identified include pain, recurrent nightmares of the accident, decreased fitness, shoulder pain in the non-involved extremity, family conflict over role changes, changing routines, and sleep disturbances. In addition, her activities have changed so much that she is struggling with her identity.

➠ What could you do to help Alice address and manage these additional problems?

➠ What community resources would assist Alice in accomplishing her goals?

➠ Summarize the recommendations you have made that would alter the treatment plan.

Let's see what happened for Alice in occupational therapy.

Alice demonstrated good initiative in implementing strategies to improve hand function and served an active role in troubleshooting and providing feedback and observations to guide the adjustments in the physical rehabilitative program. For instance, when the focus was on gaining active and passive extension, she noticed that she was beginning to have some difficulty in attaining full motion in flexion to grip. Therefore, the balance of the splinting/exercise/functional use program was adjusted to ensure ability to attain full hand motion in both flexion and extension. The therapist and client worked collaboratively to practice strategies for managing her home schedule and family needs and organization, including practical concerns, such as diapering her infant. One of her sisters spent a week at her house to assist her when she came home from the hospital. Since then, her church and neighbors have provided babysitting during therapy appointments and have assisted with grocery shopping, thus enabling her husband to continue to work his farm. The primary focus thus far has been primarily on improving hand function and implementing strategies to manage home and family. Simulation of targeted job components is incorporated into an exercise program, and a worksite visit is pending. Alice expresses confidence in her ability to manage her home and family and is pleased with her progress to this point and in her potential to resolve remaining issues and attain her goals.

Meet Annie, Bernice, and Mary Waters

The second practice situation is complicated by the structure and function of the family. It requires us to think beyond the specific needs of a person and to look at that person in a family unit, a social unit, and in society in general. Homelessness is a problem that affects more and more families. This family has problems that can benefit from an occupational therapist taking a family-systems approach to its resolution. Meet Annie, Bernice, and Mary Waters.

Annie is a 4-year-old African-American girl who has cerebral palsy (mild spastic right hemiplegia). She lives in a transitional homeless shelter apartment complex with her 20-year-old single mother, Bernice, and her 6-year-old sister, Mary. Prior to becoming homeless, they lived with her two uncles and her grandmother. Annie's grandmother visits regularly on the weekends. Her mother is in a welfare-to-work program. She currently is being trained to work as a chambermaid at a local motel and also is working to get her high school diploma. Bernice is overwhelmed by her responsibilities and says that Annie is an angel; her sister Mary, however, never stops moving and is always in trouble with her first-grade teacher. Mary attends the after-school latchkey program at the homeless shelter. Annie is enrolled in the day care program at the shelter. The family will be able to live at the homeless shelter for a total of 12 months. They have already been there for 2 months. Annie will be able to remain at the day care 1 additional year after the family leaves the homeless shelter.

Annie is referred to your agency, which provides direct occupational therapy to children at city day cares and consultative services to the classroom teachers. The day care director informs you that Annie failed her First Steps screening (as per reference) in the motor area and was "at risk" in the area of cognition. You observe Annie at her inner-city day care, which is located at the homeless shelter. You meet the recently hired teacher who had worked in a nursing home with elderly clients prior to this job. There are 15 other children in the classroom, one of whom has Down syndrome. The children range in age from 3 to 4 years of age. There is one teacher's aide, who has raised 12 children and nine grandchildren. She informs you that she "knows how to raise children."

Occupational Performance Issues

An informal 5-minute discussion with the teacher, Mrs. Johnson, reveals that she is trying to do her best for Annie. She has never seen a child quite like her before. "We treat her just like any other child in this classroom." When asked what her daily lesson plans focus on, Mrs. Johnson informs you that it is her job to teach the children their colors, shapes, numbers, and letters. When asked how she would like you to help her with Annie, she replies, "Her arm don't work quite right. Maybe you could work on it." The teacher states that the mother appears to be caring, but is always exhausted. Bernice was glad to hear that a therapist was going to work with Annie. She drops off Annie at 6:00 a.m. and picks her up at 6:00 p.m. 5 days a week.

You observe that Annie returns from the bathroom and requests that the teacher fasten and adjust her clothes. Her shoes are untied. At breakfast she encounters difficulty scooping the cereal into her bowl and pouring the milk accurately. She has difficulty scooping the cereal into her spoon. During a coloring and gluing task, Annie becomes easily frustrated, tearing most of her project. During free time, she was observed to play by herself, enjoying the "house" area, with dolls and kitchen props. She W-sits (knees in and feet out in the shape of a "W") on the floor to play. She became very absorbed in her activity and refused to put the toys away when free time was over. Snack time was similar to breakfast, where she had difficulty pouring the juice and spreading peanut butter on crackers. The teacher called the class together and drilled the children in the alphabet letters. Annie sat quietly, listened, but did not know any letters other than "A." Lastly, you observe Annie outdoors. She again plays off by herself, falling frequently, and trying unsuccessfully to maneuver a tricycle. Her right arm postures slightly in flexion. Her right leg postures in flexion and adduction. You spend a few minutes talking to Annie at recess after she seems comfortable around you. She seems eager to please, and you spend a few more minutes helping her to pedal the tricycle.

➡ What additional information do you need to have a clear understanding of the issues facing Annie, Bernice, Mary, and the teacher?

The Initial Approach to Assessment

Initial observations indicate that Annie is experiencing some difficulty with occupational performance, particularly in areas of self-care and school activities. It is hypothesized that Annie's developmental problems may be influenced by difficulty with achieving stability to perform bilateral activities. Another concern focuses on her limited social interaction, which could be influenced by her living situation or play deficits.

The main theoretical approach used is developmental, to determine her current functional status and provide age-appropriate activities. A secondary theoretical approach used by the occupational therapist is neurointegrative based on the presenting right hemiplegia. You would like to rule out any secondary perceptual deficits that may be contributing to her developmental delays.

➡ What would be the advantage of employing a person-environment-occupation model in this case?

As a result of these observations, you decide to return and formally evaluate Annie using several assessment tools. You hypothesize that Annie is having developmental problems because of difficulty achieving stability to perform bilateral self-care and classroom/developmental activities due to the right (R) hemiplegia. You would like to rule out any secondary visual perceptual problems based on your knowledge of hemiplegia, which could add to her performance deficits. Another concern focuses on her limited social interaction skills with peers.

On the Peabody Developmental Motor Scales, Annie scores at the 66th percentile, with considerable difficulties in the areas of eye-hand coordination and manual dexterity. The Test of Visual Perceptual Skills (Non-motor) indicates difficulties in visual memory and spatial relations, form constancy, figure-ground, and closure. On the Preschool Playscale, Annie is functioning at an overall age of 41.25 months, with specific limitations in the areas of gross motor activity, interest, and space management. Her strengths at age level are in the areas of construction, purpose, attention, material management, language, and participation. On the Pediatric Evaluation of Disability Inventory, Annie exhibits decreases in function in the areas of self-care, mobility, and social function.

No modifications are done currently for self-care, mobility, or social function.

In addition to these developmental assessments, you take a neurointegrative approach to assess tonal distribution, range of motion, and the presence of equilibrium and protective reactions in Annie's arm and leg. These underlying performance component issues may contribute to her lack of bilateral skills and her frequent falls.

You discover mild spasticity in elbow flexors, forearm pronators, wrist flexors, and finger flexors. Active assistive range of motion is slightly limited in elbow extension, forearm supination, wrist extension, and finger extension. Annie can only extend her wrist to neutral. She has minimal protective extension in the right arm and does not use the arm for balance during sitting or standing equilibrium. The right leg has mild spasticity in the hip internal rotators, knee extensors, and ankle plantar flexors. She has full passive range of motion, with the exception of a slight contracture in the ankle. The knee becomes hyperextended during ambulation.

These results demonstrate that Annie is far below age expectancy for self-care, mobility, and social function, which accurately reflects further findings. She lacks confidence on play structures and uneven terrains. She has not yet developed cooperative play skills with peers. Annie is struggling with tasks that require bilateral manipulation of objects and adequate standing balance due to her hemiplegia. She has difficulty cutting with scissors. She has a superior pincer grasp and is able to hold a pencil in a tripod grasp. Emerging dexterity skills include stringing beads, lacing shoes, and buttoning 3/4-inch buttons by stabilizing against body with right arm. Several visual perceptual deficits could also be contributing to her performance difficulties.

Use this information to create an occupational performance profile for Annie. If pieces are missing, identify additional questions that require answers before you would proceed as if this were a real experience.

Annie's Strengths

- Person
  - She is eager to please. Neither receptive nor expressive languages are impaired. Annie is able to communicate well enough to have her basic needs met and to stand up for herself around other children, for example, if they grab her toy.
  - Additional information/questions?
- Environmental
  - The family has located an agency that will provide for their needs for 1 full year and will provide for Annie for 1 additional year. The mother is receiving training in job readiness, living skills, and education. The maternal grandmother is still involved, although not wanting Bernice to live with her any longer. Extended family is important to Bernice and she has their support. Though Bernice is occupied for 12 hours a day with all of her own programs, she is trying to improve herself for her children.
  - Additional information/questions?
- Occupational
  - Annie is a vivacious child with adults. She is currently around 14 other children who can assist her in developing her play skills. She receives breakfast and lunch at the day care. She is toilet-trained, can follow directions, listens quietly when told, and is very polite.
  - Do we know what Annie likes to do?

Annie's Limitations

- Person
  -
- Environmental
  -
- Occupational
  -

Treatment Goals

The following treatment goals were set:

- Using adaptive equipment, Annie will be independent in age-appropriate self-care activities.
- In a play group of three children, Annie will demonstrate cooperative play interactions.
- With adaptations, Annie will be able to pedal a tricycle independently.
- What and who will be the focus of your treatment plan?

In a family-centered approach, the client is Annie and her family but, when placing the family in the context of community services, there is also the day care staff with whom the occupational therapist is consulting. This will influence the goals and the program plan that follow. The focus of these goals will be to adapt activities and promote developmental competence for Annie. What are additional issues that must be considered in building the treatment plan?

- Address how you will determine the parent's goals.

- The teacher's goals.

- Annie's goals.

- How can we support Bernice in acquiring skills to enrich the environment for her children?

- How can we support the teacher in creating a learning environment to help Annie achieve her potential?

- What role does Mary (the 6-year-old sister) play in Annie's program?

- What additional community resources would assist this family in managing their issues?

- Summarize your recommendations and ideas for the treatment plan for Annie.

Now, let's see what actually happened during occupational therapy treatment for Annie.

Focus of Direct Therapy with Annie

Focusing on the first goal with Annie, she currently requires assistance in bilateral self-care activities such as clothing adjustment after toileting, and eating activities such as pouring, scooping, and spreading. Because Annie can only extend her wrist to neutral, you explore making a functional splint, which reinforces wrist extension to improve her use of the right hand as a more effective stabilizer. You bring in some "dress-up" outfits that have pants with various kinds of fasteners. You and Annie spend time practicing with the dress-up clothes with different fastening challenges as her proficiency improves. You make brightly contrasting zipper pulls for the teacher to put on Annie's pant zippers on days when she comes to the day care with zippered pants. The color contrast helps her identify the zipper pull. You and Annie also practice each time she goes to the bathroom, fastening and adjusting her clothing. Though suggestions could be made to the mother about type of clothing she could purchase (elasticized waists and Velcro closures), this is not financially feasible for the family at this time. For all of the children in the classroom, the occupational therapist suggests simple string knot tying activities, "home-made" lacing cards, and stringing Cheerios as beginning shoe-tying activities. Through practice, developmentally appropriate activities, and a few environmental adaptations, Annie will be assisted in acquiring self-care independence.

The same approach would be taken with her eating skills. For eating proficiency, Annie requires practice and a few environmental adaptations. You supply the teacher with a few Dycem squares to be placed under her bowl and cup to prevent sliding. A heavyweight bowl and cup and a lightweight milk pitcher with spout and handle may help the situation, if they can be supplied. For pouring and scooping practice, you suggest to the teacher a sensory cardboard box filled with birdseed and assorted bottles and scoops which Annie and her classmates could use. These supplies would assist Annie in her second goal of playing around other children. For this activity, children share tools and enjoy playing next to each other but do not have a common goal to their play activities.

Each time you come to the day care, you bring a novel activity for Annie and two or three other children to work with. The focus of the play group is to work on sharing, beginning communication, and common goals. Activities, such as decorating a large cardboard box, dancing with colorful scarves, or making peanut butter playdough will all reinforce group play skills for Annie. Lastly, you adapt one of the tricycles for Annie to enhance her ability to pedal independently. A built-up pedal and a built-up handle help. You also add an abductor wedge to the right side to keep her hip in neutral. It takes a few days of practice for Annie to pedal downhill. In the classroom, to discourage W-sitting, Annie is given a stool 6 inches off the ground to sit on during circle time. In order to achieve some stretch to the right ankle, you instruct the teacher's aide how to position Annie's leg and do an assisted range of movement exercise to the song "I'm a little teapot" during circle time.

Consultative Role with Family and Day Care Staff

Staff goals relate to increasing staff knowledge about cerebral palsy, developmental activities, and providing a safe environment for Annie. The following is the plan for the consultative collaborative effort. In a consultative role, the focus of occupational therapist, developed collaboratively with Ms. Mary, will be to support the environment in order that the day care and family may promote Annie's developmental competence.

- Provide in-service training to day care teachers, focusing on developmental activities, which are precursors to letter and number recognition, including pre-literacy activities. Other topics would need to be identified by the staff and may include discipline and behavioral management techniques, toilet training, and play development.
- Locate community resources to assist with the acquisition of needed classroom supplies. The outdoor play area only has a slide, with no hand railings for the steps. Annie's classmates frequently play on this one piece of equipment. With precarious balance and a lot of other children around her, Annie is unsafe on this piece of equipment. You work with Annie, teaching her to go up the stairs by sitting on them. You also work with the day care director about safety and fundraising issues. You explore the possibility of writing a grant together to obtain needed funds.
- Assist Bernice in locating needed services for Annie, and possibly her sister, as the family transitions into a new residence and school district within 10 months.
- Talk to the after-school latchkey program personnel to see how Annie's sister is doing in that program.

Though Annie is the client, she attends day care 12 hours a day, and in this environmental context her performance needs to be supported. Though she lives with her mother, at this time it does not appear that the mother has the energy required to add anything extra to her daily routine. However, the therapist will contact the mother and meet with her, on a weekend day if necessary.

It may be possible to also engage the maternal grandmother. The focus of the family involvement would be to reinforce the self-care independence with the adaptive equipment, and to possibly carry out two passive range of motion/positioning recommendations on a daily basis.

Outcomes of Intervention

Environmental adaptations helped Annie compensate for some loss in dexterity. Annie was able to be independent in caring for all of her needs by predominantly using her left hand. The right upper extremity became more adept at stabilizing during bilateral tasks. It was, however, an ongoing effort for the aide to locate the equipment that Annie required for improved performance. Both the teacher and the aide agreed that Annie's performance was improved with the equipment. The splint was kept in the classroom after the third replacement splint was made. Bernice found it difficult to remember to bring the splint with Annie to day care each day.

The teachers enjoyed watching all of the activities that the occupational therapist did each week with Annie and her play group. They thought they were all good ideas and began to incorporate some of the cooperative play ideas into the classroom. They also continued with drills in letter and number recognition. The teacher felt that Annie was better integrated into the class, choosing activities that other children were playing, particularly the children who had been in her play group. Bernice reports that Annie would leave the apartment now to play with other children in the halls of the complex. Reassessment through observation using the Preschool Playscale confirmed that Annie's play skills were now age appropriate. Active wrist range of motion is increased to 25 degrees of extension. Passive range of movement at the ankle is within normal limits now. Annie can ride her tricycle competently on the playground, although sometimes she has difficulty going up the hill.

In Chapter Three, we have begun to consider the occupational therapy care plan and how it is developed. We will continue this in Chapter Four.

References

Law, M. (Ed.). (1998). *Client-centered occupational therapy*. Thorofare, NJ: SLACK Incorporated.

Resources

First Steps: Screening Test for Evaluating Preschoolers. Lucy Miller. (1993). The Psychological Corporation, 555 Academic Court, San Antonio, TX 78204-2498.

Peabody Developmental Motor Scales. Rhona Folio & Rebecca Fewell. (1983). The Riverside Publishing Co., 425 Spring Lake Drive, Itasca, IL 60143.

Pediatric Evaluation of Disability Inventory. PEDI Research Group. (1992). Department of Rehabilitation Medicine, New England Medical Center Hospital, #75K/R, 750 Washington Street, Boston, MA 02111-1901.

Preschool Playscale. Knox, S. (1997). Development and current use of the Know Preschool Play Scale. In D. Parham & L. Fazio (Eds.), *Play: A clinical focus in occupational therapy for children*. St. Louis, MO: Mosby-Year Books.

Test of Visual Perceptual Skills. Morrison F. Gardner. (1982). Psychological and Educational Publications, Inc., P.O. Box 520, Hydesville, CA 95547.

Notes

Notes

Section Two

Reconfiguring Our Practice

As mentioned in the description of the purpose of this book, health care professionals have faced, and continue to face, exceptional circumstances at this, the beginning of the 21st century. There is no doubt that the occupational therapy profession is in an ideal position to realize the importance of its central mission. However, in order for this to occur, there has to be a profession-wide commitment to developing a proactive position for occupational therapy. We have to be ready to recognize the need for change, and then to change. By learning from this book, you have illustrated your interest in doing this on a personal level. In the United States, Canada and other countries, there has been a commitment at national levels to support and encourage occupational therapy practitioners to adopt a forward-thinking model for practice into the new century. By moving on to the following two chapters in this section, you will be offered the opportunity to begin to work through the practical steps toward making those shifts.

Chapter Four

From Diagnosis to Occupational Performance

Carolyn M. Baum, PhD, OTR/L, FAOTA

Practice Scenario Authors: Seanne Wilkins, PhD, OT(c)
Carol DeMatteo, MSc, OT(c)

Occupational therapists' unique contribution to society is to enable clients to achieve their goals by helping them overcome problems that limit their occupational performance (Baum & Law, 1997). To achieve this goal, the practitioner learns about the clients' physical, cognitive, neurobehavioral, and psychological capacities; their culture; their physical, social, and institutional environments; and the activities, tasks, and roles that the clients define as important (Law, Cooper, Strong, Stewart, Rigby, & Letts 1997).

Some of the environments in which we work as occupational therapists make it more difficult to practice in a client-centered manner and focus on occupational performance issues. Let's explore one such environment.

Meet Sara

Sara Wilson was born at 27 weeks gestation at a local hospital. At birth, she required cardiac compressions and intubation to sustain her life. Her Apgar scores (appearance, pulse, grimace, activity, and respiration) were one at 1 minute, six at 5 minutes, and nine at 10 minutes. Her birth weight was 1.085 kg. Sara was transferred to the neonatal intensive care unit (NICU) at a medical center in a distant city. Cranial ultrasound on day 1 noted a large left subpendymal hemorrhage and intraventricular hemorrhage with slight dilatation at the left lateral ventricle. Bilateral flare was noted with serious concern for periventricular leukomalacia (PVL). The retinal exam noted zone II, stage 1 retinopathy in her left eye and stage 0 in her right eye. Sara remained ventilated for 2 months and then on low-flow oxygen and was discharged with oxygen. At 4 months, still on low-flow oxygen and on tube feedings, she was discharged back to her local hospital.

Sara is the first child of Mary and John Wilson. John works full-time shifts in a local manufacturing plant. Mary had been working at a local office, but she is not returning to her work. They purchased their first home recently. John's parents, Gladys and Harold Wilson, are very supportive and have been transporting Sara's mother to the hospital. They are willing to do anything to help.

When Did Occupational Therapy Enter the Case?

An occupational therapy consultation was requested when Sara was 1 month old. The neonatologist suspected that there may be developmental problems due to the risks of PVL. She also was extremely premature and showed evidence of an orthopedic problem with her right ankle and hip.

➠ What do you think are the most important issues for occupational therapy assessment and intervention for Sara?

Issues

The therapist interviewed the parents and grandparents, and observed Sara. She also spoke to the nursing staff and lactation consultants, and consulted with the neonatologists, nutritionists, and respiratory therapists. Sara was observed with and without her family. The therapist worked with Sara, doing handling and direct evaluation using Neonatal Individualized Developmental Care Assessment (NIDCAP) and a behavioral feeding assessment, the Neonatal Oral Motor Assessment Scale (NOMAS). The following issues were identified concerning Sara:

- Sara has limited ability to move and play as needed for her age in order to advance her development. Sara's obvious right-sided increase in tone and delay in motor skills contribute to this. Sara desaturates and becomes very distressed with any touch or movement. This interferes with and affects the approach to therapeutic, developmental, and parental interaction. Sara's over-reactivity to any sensory stimuli causes this.
- Feeding: Sara's mother is unsure but feels she should breastfeed her daughter. She is from out of town, so this will be difficult. In addition, Sara has gross incoordination, respiratory difficulties, and oral aversion. However, the staff of the NICU support breastfeeding and have been reluctant to offer her a bottle. Sara currently has nasogastric feeds through an in-dwelling tube.
- Parent-Child interaction: Sara's mother is extremely anxious and fearful of disturbing Sara at all in case she goes bradycardic or apneic. She is afraid to change her position, hold her, or move her. Right now, she does very little to the baby and just stares at her. Her mother is also exhausted. Chronic lung disease is affecting all and any interactions and interventions. The mother quickly becomes distressed, requiring increased oxygen. Sara's unstable medical status affects all performance.
- Parental roles: Interrupted due to hospitalized and chronically ill infant.

Approach

➠ Identify the performance components (intrinsic factors) that are influencing Sara's performance.

➠ Identify the environmental factors (extrinsic factors) that are influencing Sara's performance.

Client's Goals

➠ Parent's goals
 - ✧ Discharge to home
 - ✧ If the above is not possible, then discharge to local hospital
 - ✧ Sara will eat without a tube
 - ✧ Sara will develop and grow normally

➠ What would you do with Sara, her parents, and others in the NICU to achieve these goals?

Let's see what happened. The occupational therapist's plan included the following strategies:

Plan

- Occupational therapist visits will coincide with parents' visits as much as possible.
- Parents and occupational therapists will decide together what they will work on at each session. Options include breastfeeding/bottlefeeding, touching and handling in ways to increase Sara's tolerance, holding, head control, eye tracking, hands to midline positions, equipment, and toys for play.
- Educational and written materials will be provided at the time and in the manner that the parents find useful. These will include pamphlets of all pictures, no words; video tapes of sessions with Sara; and articles.
- Discharge planning with the family for all eventualities, including home or to the local hospital. Work with the family to prepare them for referral to the long-term children's rehabilitation facility. This will include decisions about home care, oxygen tube feeding, access to therapy, return for outpatient follow-up, and parent support.

➡ Which aspects of this plan focus on occupational performance, performance components, or the environment? Identify each below.

Therapy Context

The above interventions occur within the context of a very stressful environment for baby, parents, and staff. It is a life or death situation for a long period of time. There is little privacy, and the health and concerns of families are very open to others. It is a very busy and crowded environment. The philosophy is to try to do what is best for the infant and family while causing the least amount of stress. The context also includes a number of different philosophies of care and a lack of understanding of client-centered care. There are many health professionals that will interact with the family over a long period of admission. There is also the strong focus on the here and now and technology, leaving the future as a big unknown. This often becomes a shock for families. Within all of the above, there is the overriding demand and pressure to clear the beds as quickly as possible to make room for the next sick infant.

Outcomes of Intervention

1. Sara tolerated increased handling, holding, and movement without desaturating and having bradycardia.
2. Mother would actually touch and hold Sara during visits.
3. Sara began to bring her hands to midline without assistance.
4. Sara began visually tracking faces and objects for 60 degrees across midline.
5. Sara was discharged with a follow-up plan for therapy at the interim hospital, follow-up with infant development and children's treatment centers post discharge from hospital.
6. Outcome of good feeding did not happen until Sara returned as an outpatient.

➡ Which of these outcomes are occupational performance outcomes? Which of these outcomes are changes in components or environments that contribute to occupational performance?

In many cases, a medical problem may be limiting occupational performance, but in others there may not be a specific condition that is causing the difficulty. Rogers (1982) argues convincingly that through the emphasis on disease and functional deficit rather than occupational performance and competence, the biomedical influences on traditional health care have been a limiting factor in the development of occupational therapy (and its measurement methods).

In this practice situation we hope to explore the unique value of the occupational therapist in improving the health and well-being of an individual who could have easily fallen through the cracks in both the medical and social system. The client has a concerned son and a physician who recognizes that she has needs—and that occupational therapy can address those needs.

Mrs. Mary Charles

Mrs. Charles is a 75-year-old woman whose husband of 51 years has just died. Mr. and Mrs. Charles have lived in their two-story home in a small town (population: 1,500) in southern Ontario since their marriage. Their son, who is 50 years old, lives about a 2-hour drive away. Mr. Charles had severe rheumatoid arthritis. In the last year before his death, Mr. Charles had been diagnosed with cancer and had undergone extensive surgery to his face and neck. It was during surgery to rebuild his jaw that he died. Because of his rheumatoid arthritis, Mr. Charles had not worked for many years. Mrs. Charles has never worked outside the home. Mr. Charles continued to drive and took Mrs. Charles shopping, to the bank, and to collect the mail.

Over the past 5 years, Mr. and Mrs. Charles had stopped seeing friends, and their only social contacts were with family. They had also stopped travelling to their son's house for visits. Because of his pain, Mr. Charles was often "difficult." When he was feeling well, they would play cards or watch television. Over the past 6 months since his surgery for cancer, he had become increasingly depressed about his situation. He did not talk much but sat in the living room in his favorite chair and often slept for long periods throughout the day.

In the past couple of years, Mrs. Charles has complained of loss of energy, general fatigue, and tiredness. She has had difficulty rising from a chair and reports being unsteady on her feet. She has difficulty going up the stairs to her bedroom on the second floor, often crawling on her hands and knees to prevent herself from falling. A thorough medical examination with her family doctor revealed no medical reasons for her failing health. While her family doctor believes that Mrs. Charles is displaying depressive symptoms, he is reluctant to prescribe medication. He believes these symptoms are related to her recent bereavement. He will continue to monitor her mental health status. Her son is concerned about her ability to manage on her own. Because of the concerns expressed by her son, her family doctor has made a referral to occupational therapy for assessment and intervention as needed.

During the initial interview with Mrs. Charles in her home, the occupational therapist conducted an unstructured interview to gain some understanding of Mrs. Charles' current situation. Mrs. Charles talked about her husband's 40 years of suffering with rheumatoid arthritis and of the pain that he had endured. She also talked about the last year of his life in which he was diagnosed with cancer. While he had never been much of a "talker," he had hardly talked at all during the last 6 months of his life. "He had given up hope that he would ever get better and was waiting to die." His death "was a blessing because now he is no longer suffering from pain"—the pain of his arthritis and the pain following his surgery for cancer. Over the years as his arthritis left him with badly deformed hands and feet, Mrs. Charles had managed their household: preparing the meals, grocery shopping, cleaning, doing yard maintenance, and managing their finances. While Mrs. Charles drove their car, until the last few months of his life, Mr. Charles insisted on driving—"He never let me drive when he was in the car." The Cancer Society had driven him to the medical center in the nearest city for his cancer treatment. She drove the car in town but not on the highway. Now her role of caregiver is over and she feels that she cannot sit at home by herself or she will feel sorry for herself. She needs "to get out of the house and begin to do things again," but she is weak, has poor endurance, and does not trust her mobility. She also has limited her interaction with friends and neighbors.

The Canadian Occupational Performance Measure (COPM) was used to assist Mrs. Charles in identifying her occupational performance issues. During the administration of the COPM, the following issues were identified and priorities established:

1. Maintaining independence in order to remain in her own home and continue to use the second-level bedroom.
2. Getting out more socially, visiting neighbors and friends, "rather than sitting around the house feeling sorry for myself."
3. Walking uptown to get the mail, go to the hairdresser, and pick up small grocery items.
4. Visiting her son and his family for Christmas.

In a telephone call to the occupational therapist, Mrs. Charles' son indicated the following concerns:

- Her ability to remain in her own home safely.
- Her obvious failing health, which had no medical basis.
- That she might move her bedroom to the main floor room that had served as her husband's bedroom for many years.

He also relayed his wife's thoughts that his mother would improve now that his father had died and she could begin to take care of and think about herself.

➡ What additional information do you need to have a clear understanding of Mrs. Charles' situation? How would you collect the information? (Remember sensory and memory changes that may be present due to her age.)

Mrs. Charles' Personal Strengths

- Determination to continue living independently in her own home.
- Determination to get on with her life, get out more now that she no longer has to care for her husband.
- Open to discussing issues with others and the occupational therapist.
- Willing to accept suggestions from others if it will help her in the long run.
- Aware of her own feelings about the death of her husband and openly discusses these.
- Aware of importance of spiritual aspects to her life.
- Sense of humor.

Mrs. Charles' Resources

- Very supportive family who live close by, including her own brothers and sisters as well as her husband's siblings
- Very supportive son and daughter-in-law
- Lived in town all her life and knows many people
- Concerned neighbors, some young friends
- Financially secure

Begin to make a list of Mrs. Charles' strengths and limitations. If some of the information you need is not available, be sure it is addressed in the assessment area above.

➡ Mrs. Charles' Strengths

✧ Person

✧ Environmental

✧ Occupational

➡ Mrs. Charles' Limitations

✧ Person

✧ Environmental

✧ Occupational

➡ Describe how you will integrate Mrs. Charles' goals into a treatment plan.

➠ What factors will go into your treatment plan?

✧ Functional Issues

✧ Intrinsic factors: psychological issues, physiological issues, cognitive Issues, musculoskeletal issues

✧ Extrinsic factors: social, societal (payment), cultural, physical environment

Let's see what further assessment by the occupational therapist determined:

The performance components (intrinsic factors) and the environmental conditions (extrinsic factors) contributing to the occupational performance issues were identified using physical rehabilitative, environmental, and psycho-emotional approaches. Assessments included:

* Activities of daily living and instrumental activities of daily living assessments, including informal observation of performance components.
* Home assessment including potential safety issues.
* Physical evaluation, including muscle strength, coordination, balance, standing tolerance, and walking endurance, as well as the ability to climb stairs.
* The Geriatric Depression Scale. If an occupational therapy assessment had been initiated before the death of Mrs. Charles' husband, an assessment of caregiver burden might have been useful, such as the Zarit Burden Interview.

The performance components and environmental conditions contributing to the occupational performance issues follow:

* Self-care: Maintaining independence in order to remain in own home and continuing to use second-level bedroom. This seemed related to her depressive symptoms, which may have been the result of caregiver burden and social isolation. The manifestations included her complaints of general fatigue, tiredness, and loss of energy. Her unsteady gait, difficulty rising from a chair, and difficulty going upstairs was related to general deconditioning with some general muscle weakness, poor balance, lack of standing tolerance, and poor walking endurance. A referral was made to a physical therapist for general conditioning exercises, stair climbing, and increased walking tolerance. Mrs. Charles wished to continue using her bedroom on the second level because of its proximity to the main bathroom with the bathtub and shower. The main-floor bathroom included only a toilet and sink. Grab bars had been installed in the second-floor bathroom to assist Mr. Charles with self-care when his arthritis had worsened. Mrs. Charles uses the grab bars to get into the bathtub to have a shower. She does manage to go upstairs safely, although she will go up on her hands and knees if fatigued. There is a railing on the stairs, and the stairs are very narrow so she can support herself using the railing and the wall. She wears tie-up shoes with rubber soles and heels. Laundry facilities are located in the main-floor sunroom off the kitchen. Access to the house includes two steps with a railing. Other than the stair climbing, there are no other safety concerns. She is independent in all other areas of self-care including dressing, eating, hygiene, toileting, etc. She does prepare her own meals, but she lacks interest in preparing meals and shopping for one. She is confident driving in town but not on more major roads.
* Productivity: Walking uptown to get the mail, going to the hairdresser, and picking up small grocery items. Her difficulty is related to her poor general physical condition. The post office, hairdresser, and grocery store are all located on the main street, which is a three-block walk from Mrs. Charles' house. With increased functional mobility, she will be able to increase her tolerance for walking the distance there and back and carrying small packages. She will use a shopping cart on wheels if she has larger, heavy parcels to carry. She drives the car to do a major shopping trip once every 2 weeks.
* Leisure: Getting out more socially, visit neighbors and friends, "rather than sitting around the house

feeling sorry for myself." Mrs. Charles had become very socially isolated over the past few years because of her husband's disability and in the past few months because of his cancer. She no longer attends church. She does not belong to any organized groups but is aware that there is a widows' group at the local Legion. She enjoys playing cards with family. She is an avid reader and enjoys music. She plays the piano.

- Visiting her son and his family for Christmas. Her son has invited her to come to his place for Christmas (which is in 4 months). Over the past 5 years, she and Mr. Charles had stopped driving to visit their son. Although she drives in town, she is not comfortable driving on the highway or that far. She would like to be able to travel by train, but in her current physical condition she would not be able to board the train and carry a small suitcase.

In summary, performance components and environmental conditions contributing to the occupational performance issues are the need to increase general strength, endurance, and functional mobility within her home and community and the need to increase social contacts and a support network within her community.

➡ How do we as occupational therapists work with families? What is our responsibility to them, particularly when they are not located in the same area as the client?

➡ What community resources would assist Mrs. Charles in managing to live independently?

➡ Summarize your recommendations into a treatment plan for Mrs. Charles:

Let's go back to the practice scenario and see what happened with Mrs. Charles:

Client's Goals

Mrs. Charles identified occupational performance issues and priorities for their attention during the administration of the COPM. The following goals are based on those issues and priorities:

1. Maintaining independence in order to remain in own home and continuing to use second-level bedroom: Mrs. Charles will increase her ability to climb the stairs with ease within 2 weeks.
2. Getting out more socially, visit neighbors and friends, "rather than sitting around the house feeling sorry for myself": Mrs. Charles will increase her social contacts in the community within 2 months.
3. Walking uptown to get the mail, go to the hairdresser, and pick up small grocery items: Mrs. Charles will walk uptown to do errands and carry back small parcels within 6 weeks.
4. Visiting her son and his family for Christmas: Mrs. Charles will travel independently to her son's home for Christmas in 4 months.

Plan

In collaboration, Mrs. Charles and the occupational therapist developed a plan to accomplish her goals.

(1. and 3.) The occupational therapist referred Mrs. Charles to a physical therapist for conditioning exercises, to increase her walking tolerance and stair-climbing abilities. The occupational therapist helped Mrs. Charles develop a walking plan in which she increased the distance, number of errands undertaken, and carrying of parcels.

The occupational therapist introduced Mrs. Charles to work simplification and energy conservation techniques that she could use at home to help reduce her fatigue. The occupational therapist discussed meal planning with Mrs. Charles and helped her with meal planning and shopping.

(2.) Mrs. Charles contacted one of her neighbors about joining her on her daily walk. She also contacted the woman who had mentioned a widows' self-help group which meets in the town, to find out more about the group: the goals of the group, when and where they meet, and how she goes about joining the group.

(4.) Mrs. Charles and the occupational therapist worked out a plan for the trip to her son's. Mrs. Charles needed to drive to a nearby town to catch the train. This required gaining some confidence in driving on more major roads. This was accomplished through taking two or three driving lessons with the local driving school, which offers a program that focuses on safety and changes associated with aging for drivers 55 years and older. Mrs. Charles and the occupational therapist visited the train station to assess the environment for parking, stairs, walking distances, and train boarding procedures. Mrs. Charles determined what size and kind of suitcase she was able to manage. Mrs. Charles contacted the train company to find out what assistance was available to her when taking the train. She made the necessary arrangements to prearrange this assistance.

Outcomes of Intervention

The outcomes of the intervention were that Mrs. Charles is now able to climb the stairs to her second floor bedroom with confidence. Her general tolerance has increased and she is not as fatigued as previously. She states that she often takes a nap in the afternoon if she is planning to be out in the evening. She has integrated work simplification and energy conservation techniques into her daily routine of self-care and household management.

She is able to walk uptown to do some errands and carry light parcels home with her. The occupational therapist suggested that she use a cane for safety and stability during the winter months. She continues to drive her car when she does a heavy shopping trip. Her interest in preparing and eating meals on her own has increased.

She has joined the widows' self-help group, which meets once a month to provide emotional support and information about resources for instrumental support often needed by women living on their own.

She traveled to her son's by train for Christmas. She drove to the train station, left her car there, and boarded the train on her own with assistance from train personnel (he helped her get on and off the train since the step up was steep). She was able to use a small suitcase on wheels and the train personnel lifted it on and off the train for her. Her son met her at the train station and took her back to the train station for her return home. She was able to participate in all of the festivities including helping her daughter-in-law prepare dinner for 12 people. They visited friends of her son and daughter-in-law for dinner on another evening.

Mrs. Charles is very satisfied with her progress to date and feels that her relationship with the occupational therapist is beneficial. She has asked the occupational therapist to assist her in the accomplishment of some additional goals.

Mrs. Charles' siblings and son tried to encourage her to use the first-level bedroom rather than maintain her own bedroom on the second floor. While they were very direct in their attempts to persuade her of the merits of this plan, she remained adamant that she did not wish to change her bedroom. She was comfortable there. It was arranged as she liked it and close to the full bathroom, including the shower. She maintained her position on this despite their attempts to convince her to change her bedroom to the main level to avoid using the stairs.

In Chapters Three and Four we have explored some of the issues in putting together a care plan for occupational therapy services for different practice situations. In the next four chapters, we will explore specific issues that are integral to developing and implementing a client-centered, occupation-based practice. Let's move on.

References

Baum, C. M., & Law, M. (1997). Occupational therapy practice: Focusing on occupational performance. *Am J Occup Ther, 51*(4), 277-288.

Law, M., Cooper, B., Strong, S., Stewart, D., Rigby, P., & Letts, L. (1997). Theoretical contexts for the practice of occupational therapy. In C. Christensen & C. Baum (Eds.), *Occupational therapy: Enabling function and well-being* (2nd ed). Thorofare, NJ: SLACK Incorporated.

Rogers, J. C. (1982). Order and disorder in medicine and occupational therapy. *Am J Occup Ther, 36,* 29-35.

Notes

Notes

Chapter Five

Doing Client-Centered Practice

Sue Baptiste, MHSc, OT(c)

Practice Scenario Authors: Lori Letts, MA, OT(c)
Susan Stark, PhD, OTR
Muriel Westermorland, MHSc, OT(c)

Background

In this chapter, we will explore issues related to implementing a client-centered practice in occupational therapy. When we think about occupational therapy practice at its best, we often talk about the person—the client—being able to feel once more like an active participant in his or her own life. We refer to activities and occupations having "meaning" to the individual; we marvel at the tenacity of the human spirit and the amazing results and outcomes that we observe—people who accomplish astonishing things, given their physical deficits and/or deep-seated mental health problems. In summary, we, as active participants in our clients' lives, gain immense satisfaction from seeing these accomplishments and deeming ourselves to be a part of them, however small.

However, in earlier times of occupational therapy practice, we tended to frame these successes in the light of the patient (the one in need) coming to the expert (the occupational therapist) for guidance, information, and direct hands-on treatment in order to achieve such positive outcomes. As we look to re-examine our practice and to redefine a practice framework, we begin to see the basic relationship in different terms. We have begun to understand that the therapeutic mission is best served by engaging in a positive partnership, within which the client and the therapist bring their unique contributions. The therapist offers knowledge, skill, experience, and focused critical thinking. The client provides a special perspective of personal experiences, sensate knowledge of the illness or trauma, and a history of a unique lifestyle, which is his or hers alone.

Client-centeredness as a concept emerged first through the writings of Carl Rogers, a psychologist. In his book *The Clinical Treatment of the Problem Child* (1939), Rogers presented a different model for therapeutic intervention which stemmed from seeking concerns from the client in order to provide direction for therapy. Rogers stated that the role of the therapist is to assist in problem solving by supporting the individual in understanding the problems confronting him or her and thus stimulating the definition of possible solutions. He had an implicit belief in the abilities of his clients to wrestle with their life problems and, with guidance and acceptance from a non-judgmental therapist, to develop a positive plan for change and future achievement (Law, 1998).

In a client-centered approach to working with people, therapists acknowledge and celebrate the myriad of differences between individuals. They accept the lack of prescribed methodologies, recognizing that it is this openness and flexibility that enriches the therapeutic partnership.

An understanding of the core elements of client-centered practice is essential if we are to examine our current practice styles and determine whether we are functioning in a manner close or distant from a client-centered model.

For a detailed overview of the varying definitions of client-centeredness, a good resource is *Client-Centered Occupational Therapy*, edited by Law (1998); and, to quote once again directly from that text, the following list of common concepts from all models of client-centered practice is offered to provide a baseline understanding:

- Respect for clients and their families, and the choices they make.
- Clients and families have the ultimate responsibility for decisions about daily occupations and occupational therapy services.
- Provision of information, physical comfort, and emotional support. Emphasis on person-centered communication.
- Facilitation of client participation in all aspects of occupational therapy service.
- Flexible, individualized occupational therapy service delivery.
- Enabling clients to solve occupational performance issues.
- Focus on the person-environment-occupation relationship.

Who is the Client?

Having been "raised" in a climate of the medical model, it is not surprising that we, as occupational therapists, tend to begin our definition of who is our client by assuming that it is the individual who has been labeled as the "patient." For many years, we have focused our attention on the person whose name appears on the referral we have received or who occupies the room or bed within the treatment unit in which we work.

A client-centered approach to practice provides a much broader opportunity for exploring the concept of "client." Certainly, the individual who has been referred is often the primary client; however, other individuals, agencies, and so on join the network, which impacts upon and provides support to the original "patient." For example, on many occasions we find ourselves working within a complex family system. Common occurrences of this often center on clients who are either children or older adults. The caregivers are in essence clients as well.

As roles for occupational therapists have expanded over recent years, another nature of clientele has emerged. Examples of these include industry, government agencies, and third-party payers. These relationships are most often noted in situations where the occupational therapist is acting in a consultative manner to a business, company, agency, or government department.

This whole discussion presents many complex facets, most particularly those related to the potential ethical dilemmas and debates which can emerge when multiple clients identify conflicting needs and demands. It becomes imperative then that all practicing occupational therapists develop a clear understanding of the scope of their own practice, the implications for practicing within a client-centered framework, and a definition of who represents their particular clients.

Meet Mrs. Jay

Mrs. Jay is a 74-year-old woman, referred to home care for occupational therapy services. Her son, who stated that he was concerned about his mother's social isolation and her ability to remain at home safely, initiated the referral. Mrs. Jay has lived in her two-bedroom bungalow for many years. She has been a widow for 8 years, and has only one son. He and his new wife recently moved into the basement in order to care for Mrs. Jay, since she was diagnosed with Alzheimer's disease about 6 months ago.

Mrs. Jay lives in a large, urban community on a relatively quiet street. She is no longer driving her own car, and the closest bus stop for public transit is about three blocks away. She spends most of her days alone at home, since both her son and daughter-in-law work outside the home. She does not leave the house unaccompanied. She is a heavy smoker. Prior to her retirement at age 65, she worked as a department store clerk for 20 years.

Mrs. Jay's son is in his 40s, and this is his second marriage. He has a work history that is very inconsistent, with most jobs lasting no longer than 1 year. He has been known to have a quick temper and a history of verbal and physical abuse of his first wife. According to Mrs. Jay, however, he has never hit her. Financially, he has many debts; he controls his mother's money and also has his wife's pay deposited into his bank account.

➡ What do you think may be potential issues for you in proceeding with this referral?

➡ Reflect on your current occupational therapy practice: how would therapists normally proceed with defining treatment direction?

➡ Now, think of what you know about client-centered practice: how might this influence how you proceed?

Occupational Performance Issues, Using a Client-Centered Approach

Initially, identifying occupational performance issues with Mrs. Jay was quite difficult. Although she was able to communicate verbally and seemed to understand what was explained to her, she was suspicious about why the occupational therapist was there and was not willing to share information about any challenges or difficulties she was facing. The occupational therapist used the first three visits to observe Mrs. Jay at home and to discuss informally how she was managing with issues currently, as well as discussing her past experiences. The therapist also shared information about herself and her own interests. This enabled Mrs. Jay and the therapist to develop a relationship of trust so that eventually Mrs. Jay was willing to share more information. Through those initial discussions, it became clear that Mrs. Jay had difficulties with short-term memory.

Other issues could be noted through observation. Mrs. Jay's clothing and general appearance were quite unkempt, and the therapist often saw her in the same clothes. There was little food in the cupboards and the refrigerator. Mrs. Jay was not doing her own shopping and did not want to venture out alone. She was independent in dressing, bathing, and toileting, but was no longer cooking, shopping, or doing the laundry. She did report that she liked to make herself a cup of tea during the day; she is a heavy smoker and there were cigarette burns on her clothing. She said she enjoyed smoking and was unwilling to consider quitting.

She also revealed that she had some concerns about her son's motivation for moving in with her. She felt that he may have moved home so that he could move her into a nursing home and have her house to himself. She complained that he wanted her to give him power of attorney, but that she was adamant that she did not want him managing her affairs. The therapist was not certain if Mrs. Jay's fears were justified or related to her cognitive impairment.

The therapist met with the son to discuss how Mrs. Jay's bills were paid. He stated he had his mother sign checks in order to pay bills. He said it was a real ordeal because his mother was reluctant to sign. He was willing to consider having his mother's finances managed by the Office of the Public Trustee, since he said it would relieve him of the stress of trying to get his mother to sign checks and any other documents. Mrs. Jay also agreed that this was a reasonable option.

Through interviews, the therapist explored Mrs. Jay's past and current leisure interests. She enjoyed watching television, although she did comment that there were times when she felt lonely. Prior to her retirement, she often got together with co-workers to play cards, although she did state that she had never been "one to belong to organized clubs."

➡ Considering all the information so far, and reflecting on elements of client-centered practice, how would you proceed at this stage? What are the key issues emerging for Mrs. Jay?

➡ Now, try to convert these issues into goals that you feel Mrs. Jay would identify to help direct her treatment plan.

What Happened in Mrs. Jay's Relationship With Her Therapist?

First, let's consider the goals as Mrs. Jay identified them in collaboration and partnership with her therapist:

1. To remain in her own home as long as possible.
2. To ensure her personal finances are managed to support her best interests.
3. To decrease loneliness from being at home alone all day.

The process of establishing goals was challenging at times, since Mrs. Jay and her therapist did not always agree on some of the key issues of concern. This was particularly true when discussing home hazards. Mrs. Jay did not see any problems with her home set up or her smoking behavior and was unconcerned about the cigarette burns on her clothing. The therapist attributed this to some lack of insight related to her cognitive impairment and perhaps to her strong desire to remain at home. The therapist had to spend time discussing with Mrs. Jay how making her home safer would enable her to remain in her home longer and emphasized that this was the goal toward which they were both working.

The resulting treatment plan included strategies for increasing social contacts, increasing supports at home, and increasing family members' knowledge about Alzheimer's disease. Modifications were organized to the home environment in order to ensure safety.

➡ Now, considering the scope of the treatment plan, what elements would be difficult in assuming a client-centered posture with Mrs. Jay? Think about current occupational therapy practice and how it might look differently if you were working with Mrs. Jay.

Ensuring a partnership with Mrs. Jay, a client with cognitive impairment, was challenging for the occupational therapist. Mrs. Jay was encouraged to make decisions at a level at which she was deemed capable and at which she was comfortable. For example, although she may not have been able to make financial decisions, she was certainly capable of deciding what she wanted to eat for breakfast or which sweater she wanted to wear.

At other times, Mrs. Jay required extra time or reassurance to adjust to changes. For example, when a new homemaker was brought into the home, she had to be given time to get to know that person before a trusting relationship could develop. Due to her cognitive impairment, the son and daughter-in-law were also significant to the client-therapist relationship. Although they provided some support to Mrs. Jay, they made it clear that further education and links with occupational therapy were not wanted.

What Happened to Mrs. Jay?

With the supports that were put in place for her, Mrs. Jay was able to remain in her home for 2 years from the time of the initial referral. The staff and driver from the day care program that she attended observed an increased tendency for Mrs. Jay to wander away from her home, and the public trustee noted that financial resources were not available to provide Mrs. Jay with 24-hour care. Therefore, the decision was made that it would be best for Mrs. Jay to be admitted to a nursing home at that point.

Although this outcome is not surprising, it is evident that the supports put in place for Mrs. Jay enabled her to meet her occupational performance goals, and to do so in a way that sustained her for longer than might otherwise have been possible.

There were some barriers that needed to be overcome during the occupational therapy process. The initial barrier for the occupational therapist was to develop a trusting relationship with Mrs. Jay, who was quite suspicious at the beginning. This involved taking time in the first visits to get to know Mrs. Jay and to let Mrs. Jay get to know her. Standardized cognitive testing could never be completed with Mrs. Jay because of her hostility when it was attempted. The occupational therapist made the decision that it was more important for her to establish a relationship with Mrs. Jay. The therapist did manage to use standardized instruments, such as the Kitchen Task Assessment and SAFER tool, which were less threatening for Mrs. Jay. With these assessments, the therapist gained knowledge about Mrs. Jay's performance and safety issues.

Another barrier was the presence of Mrs. Jay's son and daughter-in-law. Their relationship with Mrs. Jay was not a simple one, and, although there were issues of neglect, they also played an important role for Mrs. Jay by providing her with a sense of security at night in her home. The occupational therapist did her best to provide information and education to the family, and to work with other community supports to ensure that Mrs. Jay's needs were met. Mrs. Jay faced a significant barrier herself when she began attending the day program. Although it met a number of her needs for social support, monitoring, and leisure, its location in a nursing home was difficult for her to accept and understand.

However, the key barrier was faced by the occupational therapist at the beginning of treatment. This occurred while establishing a client-centered approach to working with Mrs. Jay despite her cognitive impairment. Although she may not have been able to understand at all times the issues being debated, or the choices that were before her, the therapist was able to establish goals with Mrs. Jay. She was able to work with her, at a level appropriate to her cognitive skills, to give her choices whenever possible and to create an environment that was supportive of her abilities and wishes, while not compromising safety issues.

Who is the Client in Client-Centered Practice?

Occupational therapists, over time, have tended to see patients, and now clients, as individuals who have been identified as having problems and issues that would benefit from attention by an occupational therapist. With the advent of client-centered practice, this territory has tended to change, expand, and encompass a much broader understanding of the term, including individuals, yes, but adding family systems, community support networks, industry, private business, and government agencies.

In order to illustrate this renewed vision of our client base, we will visit the city zoo and assume the role of an occupational therapist. The therapist has been retained as the leader of a team to address issues raised from a lawsuit levied against the zoo by a group of people with disabilities. The city zoo was found to be non-compliant with the guidelines under the Americans with Disabilities Act (ADA) that require a minimum level of accessibility for all features of a government or private agency. The charge in the suit was that people with disabilities were discriminated against because the train that transported visitors around the park was not accessible. The city zoo chose to settle rather than go to court and, in the settlement negotiations, the plaintiffs stated their major concern that the zoo was not responsive to the needs of visitors with disabilities. Examples they cited included insensitivity by employees and limitations on what people with disabilities could do while at the zoo due to physical and policy barriers (e.g., those with guide dogs were asked to leave, information videos did not have closed captioning). The plaintiffs have stipulated that you (an occupational therapist with expertise in environmental modifications) be hired to lead a team mandated with bringing about the necessary changes. Members of your team include:

- Zoo administrators from human resources, grounds keeping, computer and technical services, and architectural planning.
- People with a wide range of disabilities.
- Attorneys.

Your role is to lead the team in making reasonable accommodations for the guests, identifying architectural and policy barriers under the ADA, and providing training to improve the sensitivity of zoo employees toward persons who have disabilities. The city zoo qualitatively estimates that "not many disabled people visit the zoo" and used that argument against becoming user-friendly to the population of persons with disabilities in the community.

➠ Who do you see as your client in this scenario?

Although the city zoo funds your services, your "client" in this case is really not the zoo at all. The true client will not be present for your assessment and intervention at the zoo. The "clients" include zoo visitors who have disabilities. The plaintiffs have made clear to you that they are merely representatives of the larger group of persons who function with disabilities within the community.

➠ What are the implications of having a group as a client?

➠ How would you begin to find out about the issues from your clients' perspectives?

Initially, you hold interviews with the plaintiffs in order to define the areas of key concern relative to issues of occupational performance. These were:

- Decreased social participation in all zoo activities.
- Increased environmental barriers to occupational performance.
- Negative attitudes toward people with disabilities.

➠ What other strategies could you use to gain information and further understanding of the situation?

Your approach to data collection and clarification could take many different routes:

- Interview zoo users and their caregivers.
- Discuss the individual complaints with the relevant plaintiff.
- Interview employees who had high levels of contact with the public to identify past problems and issues.
- Perform an activity audit to explore the types of activities that were possible to experience at the zoo.

An activity audit is a qualitative evaluation of all the activities for typical users of a facility that are possible within that facility. The activities are listed and an analysis is performed to identify potential physical, policy, and attitudinal barriers for persons with disabilities. The analysis is based on the Enabler Matrix (Steinfeld, et al. 1979), an environmental assessment that considers occupational performance within a context given the performance limitations of the users. From this process emerges a sense of potential occupational performance problems.

➠ Reflect on your assumptions about who the typical users of the city zoo would be.

The groups of typical users included:

- Family members
- Friends
- Naturalists
- Workers
- Students
- Volunteers

➠ What kinds of occupational performance issues would you expect to see identified (using a client-centered approach)?

Examples of the occupational performance issues that were identified as problematic prior to intervention are given here. Visitors cannot:

- Toilet independently due to architectural barriers in the restrooms.
- View the exhibits independently due to some exhibits presenting barriers to persons who have cognitive, physical, or sensory impairments.
- Purchase items from the gift shop independently because of barriers in the café.
- Participate in leisure activities independently with friends and family due to barriers.
- Move around the facility independently due to barriers.

In summary, you find that there are multiple environmental factors that contribute to the "unfriendly" nature of the city zoo. The buildings are not compliant with the minimum standards for accessibility; the attitudes of employees toward interacting with people with disabilities are negative; and the policies of the zoo, both real and perceived, have created an environment and culture that are not welcoming.

➡ How can you move ahead with your job in a client-centered manner?

➡ What strategies/actions should you utilize to develop an outcome plan?

Using a client-centered approach, you negotiate with the plaintiffs and the zoo to work with the team to develop an outcome plan that will bring the zoo into compliance with the ADA. Based on the goals of the plaintiffs, the zoo administrators, and the attorneys for both sides, the following goals are defined:

- Improved opportunity for social participation within the zoo and improved usability of the zoo by visitors with disabilities.
- Increased numbers of visits with families who have members with disabilities.
- Improved educational experiences of persons who have disabilities.
- Increased work opportunities for persons with disabilities.

What Happened at the City Zoo in the End?

Overall, there was much success achieved from the point of view of all players. All zoo employees were provided with training in creating and maintaining a collaborative and friendly environment, with some choosing to continue further. The employees felt that their knowledge and understanding were much improved. A long-term access plan was devised for the existing zoo exhibits and a policy for the review of all new construction projects was implemented. Where permanent modifications were not feasible because of cost, temporary solutions were provided. All of the originally identified barriers were accounted for in this plan.

➡ What types of barriers do you think would have existed to the development of such a collegial result?

There were many barriers to the intervention plan that you developed for the city zoo. These barriers will continue to exist as the zoo management and employees attempt to make their facility usable for visitors with disabilities. The cost of making existing exhibits accessible is considerable when attempting to plan for all types of disabilities. The technology is often not readily available for making the unique exhibits at the zoo accessible. Making a bear pit or a hands-on river exhibit accessible is sometimes a challenge for the designers, who need to account for the experience and needs of the animals as well as the visitors.

Overall, this was an intensely gratifying, if challenging, experience given the complexity of the groups of key players and the potential diversity of their special interests and needs. Occupational therapy input continues to be requested as further exhibits are planned and constructed.

Industry as Client

For the final element of this chapter, we will explore another scenario that is based in the production industry. Minimal case information is provided but is steered with key questions based on client-centered practice principles so that you can apply your learning to these issues.

You have been asked by WGX Products Ltd. (makers of health, beauty, and food products) to provide consultation in relation to their soap packaging line. They are finding that a number of their employees are complaining of repetitive strain injury, and this is affecting line productivity.

➠ Do you understand all the information in this statement?

➠ What are the learning issues for you here?

WGX is a company of 2,000 employees situated in a factory built in the early 1900s. The soap product line is up three flights of steps, with only a service elevator at the other end of the building. The company is known for having its employees work in teams and for encouraging them to solve problems on the job. The work area is fairly well lit and covers approximately 4,000 square feet. The machinery was installed in 1985, and the packing and inspection is carried out manually. Three people work on the line with the wrapping machine and three do the packing. Bundles of three bars of soap are manually taken off the line and placed in the boxes, which are made ahead of time by the packers.

You have been asked to review the occupational tasks associated with this production line, particularly the packing tasks, and to make recommendations to modify the line to prevent exacerbation of repetitive strain injury.

➠ Who is your primary client in this scenario?

➠ What issues can you foresee in developing recommendations based on a client-centered approach to occupational therapy?

➠ Who should you involve in your search for information?

➠ What strategies could you use to approach your information search in order to broadly identify the issues?

➡ What kinds of occupational performance issues would you expect to identify?

➡ What barriers do you think could emerge from your environmental scan?

➡ What recommendations would you see making to WGX regarding their potential line modifications?

➡ How would you approach your client to submit the recommendations for its consideration?

Once the central ideas underlying client-centered practice have become clear and comfortable, then the next stage is to apply them against a backdrop of real-world clinical situations within specific areas of practice to see how they work and any differences that emerge between practice settings. The next two chapters allow that opportunity.

Let's move on to Chapter Six, where we discuss the focus of occupational therapy intervention.

References

Law, M. (Ed.). (1998). *Client-centered occupational therapy.* Thorofare, NJ: SLACK Incorporated.

Rogers, C. R. (1939). *The clinical treatment of the problem child.* Boston: Houghton-Mifflin.

Steinfeld, E., Schroeder, S., Duncan, J., Faste, R., Chollet, D., Bishop, M., Wirth, P., & Cardell, P. (1979). *Access to the built environment: A review of the literature.* Washington, D.C.: U.S. Government Printing Office.

Notes

Section Three

Focusing Our Practice

This section is designed to assist the practitioner in defining the focus and outcomes of intervention. It requires us to ask questions like, Who is the client? What are his or her needs? What is the feasibility of the intervention? How do I enable the client to achieve his or her goals? How do I define the outcomes of occupational therapy?

In Chapters Six and Seven, we use case examples to explore how occupational therapists identify occupational performance issues, gather information regarding client strengths, and determine the most appropriate focus for initial occupational therapy intervention.

In Chapter Eight, discussion centers on the determination of client outcomes to enable therapists to readily identify and link occupational performance issues to expected outcomes and strategies for outcome measurement.

Chapter Six

Defining Occupational Therapy Intervention

Carolyn M. Baum, PhD, OTR/L, FAOTA

Practice Scenario Authors: Cheryl Missiuna, PhD, OT(c)
Monica S. Perlmutter, MA, OTR/L

Occupational therapists work in several different models including health promotion and disease prevention. Over the years, we have seen occupational therapy move from that of prescribed activities to one of identification of problems that require an occupational therapist intervention. This chapter will employ two practice situations: a habilitation approach and the other a rehabilitation approach. In this chapter, we will explore the process of defining the focus of intervention for both perspectives.

Habilitation involves learning, constructing experiences for growth, creating enriched environments, and providing opportunities for the client in the occupations of choice. First, Jared Williams provides us with a perspective of the occupational therapist's role in the habilitation process.

Meet Jared

Jared is 8 1/2 years old. He has recently entered grade 3 at Ridgemount Public School. Following a parent-school meeting at the end of grade 2, Jared was referred to occupational therapy through School Health Support Services due to difficulty with printing, task completion, and social isolation. At this point, the school does not plan to refer Jared for psychological or educational testing, since his academic difficulties appeared to be limited to those activities that have a motor basis.

Jared's parents are in agreement with the referral recommended by the school and have expressed additional concerns about his difficulty in getting ready for school in the mornings. Jared's parents also indicate that he has few leisure interests and does not play with other children in the neighborhood. Jared is the older child of Mr. and Mrs. Williams, a young professional couple who also have a daughter, Sarah, who is 6 years of age. Sarah is reported to be a popular child who is reading well and has many friends. Sarah takes piano lessons and attends gymnastics classes. The Williams family lives in a modest home in an urban setting and within walking distance of the public school that Jared and Sarah attend. Mr. Williams is a journalist with a local newspaper and Mrs. Williams works part-time as a nurse.

Occupational Performance Issues

The occupational therapist who received the referral contacted Mrs. Burton, Jared's teacher, and arranged a meeting to obtain information about how Jared was functioning at the end of the first month in grade 3. The occupational therapist completed a Canadian Occupational Performance Measure (COPM) (Law, Baptiste, Carswell, McColl, Polatajko, & Pollock, 1994) with Mrs. Burton. She indicated that Jared was still struggling with any task that required written output and that his work was rarely completed within class time. He has difficulty with any type of social interaction at school and does not like to participate in any games at recess or in more structured activities during physical education class. Recently, with the beginning of formal handwriting instruction, Jared has begun to demonstrate more anger and frustration in the classroom: he has torn up his workbook and pushed another child who touched him. Jared is an excellent reader and likes to do oral presentations if he is permitted to work on his own.

When the COPM was completed with Mrs. Williams, she expressed concern about Jared's ability to dress himself independently and complete the morning routine required to get ready for school. Mrs. Williams described Jared as a "couch potato" who watches a lot of television and plays computer games. He has to be forced to go outside to play and, once outside, will not engage in road hockey or ball games with neighborhood children. Jared has recently learned to ride a bicycle but is not yet proficient on rougher terrain. Mrs. Williams indicated that her husband is frustrated by Jared's self-care difficulties, expressing the belief that she does too much for Jared and babies him, but that Mr. Williams is not bothered by Jared's lack of participation in physical activities, saying, "We can't all be athletes."

After a short classroom observation, the occupational therapist met with Jared and completed a modified COPM with him. The occupational therapist reviewed a typical day with Jared, beginning with his morning routine and discussing many of the activities that would occur at school or at home. Jared expressed concern about "the stupid writing stuff" he had to do at school and about the fact that he could not catch or throw balls in order to play basketball. He indicated that he does not have any friends because he does not know how to play any of the sports that are of interest to them. He also stated that he did not like the amount of homework that he had to do and that his mother and teacher always seemed to be mad at him for forgetting something. These latter comments appeared to be related to failure to complete his work at school, thereby necessitating completion at home.

The occupational therapist hypothesized that Jared's difficulties might be related to the coordination difficulties normally associated with developmental coordination disorder. Attention and behavioral concerns also need to be investigated, as do the environmental expectations that are being placed by the teacher and parents. A developmental approach within a person-environment-occupation model will be utilized to guide the assessment process with a focus on ascertaining Jared's developmental level in fine and gross motor skill development and self-concept. Classroom observation and discussion with the teacher indicated that Jared is not functioning at the level expected of other students in grade 3 during any activity requiring motor output; the teacher's expectations do not appear to be unusual for children of this age. Jared's reading ability is reported to be at a grade 5 level.

Person-Oriented Assessments

The Bruininks-Oseretsky Test of Motor Proficiency (Bruininks, 1978), the Beery Developmental Test of Visual-Motor Integration (Beery, 1989), the Self-Perception Profile for Children (Harter, 1985), and a locally developed handwriting test were administered to Jared. The test results are presented in Tables 6-1 and 6-2.

- Bruininks—Jared's scores on the gross motor, fine motor, and full battery composite indicate that his performance is considerably below the typical performance expected for a child of this age. Fine motor items appear to be more problematic than gross motor items, with greatest difficulty seen on tasks requiring bilateral coordination and visual-motor control.
- Beery—Jared's score indicates that his ability to complete a design-copying task is very delayed for a child of his age.
- Harter—Scores range from 1 to 4, with scores below 3 indicating that the child perceives himself to be less competent than his peers on many of the items contained in that subscale.
- Additional handwriting observations:
    - "Raging bull" tendencies when frustrated (face reddens, body tenses, stomps foot or hits self with fist on lap)
    - Appeared embarrassed, stressed, agitated with difficult tasks
    - Good attention to task during listening, reading activities
    - Comprehension of verbal instructions is very good
    - Little evidence of ability to problem solve or clarify expectations with difficult tasks
    - On playground, stands alone watching other children or plays with much younger children
    - Decreased eye contact during any social interaction

The results of the standardized assessments and of the therapist's observations confirmed the hypothesis that Jared was showing characteristics that are typical of a child with developmental coordination disorder. The occupational therapist asked Mr. and Mrs. Williams to

Table 6-1 Bruininks, Harter, and Beery Test Results for Jared

Bruininks	*Standard Score*	*Harter*	*Mean*	*Beery (VMI)*	*Score*
Running speed	9	Scholastic competence	3.7	Raw score	6
Balance	10	Social appearance	2.5	Percentile	1
Bilateral coordination	4	Physical appearance	2.5	Z score	-2.3
Strength	20	Behavioral conduct	3.5	Standard score	65
Gross motor composite	43	Global self-worth	2.8		
Upper limb coordination	10	Athletic competence	2.8		
Response speed	19				
Visual-motor control	1				
Upper limb speed	17				
Fine motor composite	27				
Battery composite	37				
Percentile rank	10				
Stanine	2				

Table 6-2 Handwriting Test Results for Jared

Test		*Observations*
Grasp:	Static tripod	Awkward, tense, stopped frequently to shake his hand
Writing speed:	20 letters per minute	
Near copy:	14 letters per minute	Copied one to two letters at a time
Far copy:	12 letters per minute	Whispered letters to self
Dictation:	24 letters per minute	Able to remember three to four words
Composition:	20 letters per minute	Complete sentence for each picture

Note: Jared completed the test using printing.

have Jared reviewed by his pediatrician in order to confirm these findings and to receive a medical diagnosis of developmental coordination disorder.

Strengths of the Client and Therapist

Jared has a number of strengths and resources. He is placed in a neighborhood school in a classroom with 25 other children and a teacher who is concerned about his welfare. Mrs. Burton is willing to adapt or modify the curriculum in order to meet Jared's needs, if required. Mr. and Mrs. Williams are supportive, involved parents who are willing to act as advocates for Jared and to participate in the therapeutic process. Jared is bright, reads well, and is able to learn and retain new knowledge if it is presented orally or in written form. School personnel indicate that Jared is showing no evidence of learning disabilities or attention deficit disorder. Jared's motor skills are delayed relative to his peers, but he has achieved most acquired motor skills to the level that would be expected of about a 6-year-old child. While Jared's self-concept is low, he has only recently begun to show behavioral and emotional outbursts that may be secondary to his motor difficulties and, therefore, is likely to be amenable to intervention. The occupational therapist has about 5 years experience, is able to provide direct intervention to Jared on a weekly basis for about 3 months, and can maintain consultative involvement after that.

Summarize the formal testing and observations into the following framework:

- Jared's strengths
    - Person

✧ Environmental

✧ Occupational

Jared's limitations

✧ Person

✧ Environmental

✧ Occupational

Client's Goals

Based upon the results of the COPM and subsequent discussion with Jared, three goals have been identified:

1. Jared will demonstrate use of strategies that enable him to keep up with the class during copying and written language activities.
2. Jared will be able to throw a basketball with sufficient accuracy to go through the hoop one of three times.
3. Jared will remember to take home all of his homework each day and will bring it back to school the next day.

In pediatrics, the parent and teacher are often considered to be clients. The majority of the teacher's concerns will be addressed through the achievement of these outcomes. Jared did not acknowledge any difficulty with the morning routine during the COPM. Therefore, Mrs. Williams' concerns about this issue will be addressed through generalization of the strategies used to achieve goal 3. Specific concerns regarding socialization and failure to participate in leisure activities will be managed through education and consultation to the parents and teacher.

Plan

A brief description of the plan to address each of the client-chosen goals follows:

Jared's Plan

Jared is motivated to perform more efficiently at school because he does not like having so much homework. The majority of his homework is a result of failing to complete tasks within class time; therefore, the focus of the intervention will be upon strategies to improve Jared's ability to keep up with the class and to produce acceptable written products. A combination of cognitive and compensatory models of practice will be used to address this issue. The therapist will work with Jared on actual tasks, using questioning techniques to help Jared discover cognitive strategies for copying, organizing work on the page, letter formation (manuscript and cursive), and checking written work. Jared wishes to improve his ability to play basketball so that he can interact with children in his neighborhood after school and can participate in basketball at recess. He is also required to work on this skill during physical education class. The occupational therapist will use a cognitive approach with Jared during basketball in order to illustrate the strategies that will be useful to Jared when learning any new motor skill. Jared will learn to describe the motor plan accurately, to examine his body position prior to and during throwing the basketball, to verbally state strategies to improve the accuracy of the throw, and to evaluate each throw once completed, using the information to change his motor plan. The approach used at school to help Jared organize his desk, locker, and homework assignments will involve a combination of cognitive and compensatory strategies. Jared will learn to use a modified reminder binder to record assignments and homework. A color coding system will be used for notebooks, report covers, textbooks, the schedule on his locker door, and the binder. Questions will be used to guide Jared through the process until such time as he discovers a strategy that works. This approach will be generalized to the morning routine at home once it is being demonstrated successfully at school.

Teacher's Plan

The teacher will modify expectations of written products by allowing some material to be presented orally; he also will provide access to a keyboard for draft and final copies of longer stories or written work, require 50% of the normal repetition of newly learned cursive letters, and accept linked manuscript or printing for all spelling tests. Whenever possible, math problems and science notes will be photocopied and provided to Jared to decrease the time spent copying from the board.

Parents' Plan

Jared's parents will be asked to provide Jared with a children's keyboarding program at home and to require 10 minutes a day of practice such that Jared learns to keyboard with greater facility. In order to increase his motivation to become more familiar with the computer, the use of video games could also be encouraged; since this tends to be a solitary activity, however, they should be used in moderation. The occupational therapist will provide Jared's parents with written information about developmental coordination disorder and about cognitive approaches that may be useful to them. She will meet with them to discuss this information further, particularly with regard to self-care and leisure activities. The therapist will discuss the types of sports and community activities that are most likely to be successful for Jared and will suggest strategies for new motor learning, as well as addressing organizational and social issues. Compensatory strategies, such as the use of Velcro shoelaces, sweat suits, and adapted toothpaste holders would be suggested to decrease the stress associated with morning and bed time routines. The challenges of upcoming elementary school grades will also be shared (e.g., increased expectation for written output) in order to encourage the development of keyboarding skills. Any other concerns that Mr. and Mrs. Williams have will be discussed.

Context

The occupational therapist will work with Jared at school, conducting part of the session in a quiet setting in the classroom and part of the session in the gym or on the playground. One session will take place in Jared's home in order to establish cues and strategies for the morning routine and to address any other concerns that his parents may have. Following the 3-month period of direct intervention, the occupational therapist will be available for consultative support at the request of Jared, the teacher, and the parents.

Outcomes of Intervention

The assumption that is made with developmental coordination disorder is that the underlying motor impairment will not be changed with intervention; therefore, the focus of the evaluation of outcome will be upon measuring the effectiveness of the cognitive and compensatory strategies in addressing the issues of concern. Following 3 months of weekly intervention, the occupational therapist re-administered the COPM with Mrs. Burton, Mrs. Williams, and Jared:

- Jared was much happier with his performance at school. He was finishing the majority of work during school and was remembering to take homework home most of the time. Work done on the keyboard produced a much neater product, but it was still slow and sometimes frustrating for him. Being permitted to focus on the subject (e.g., math, spelling, and science) rather than the type or neatness of the writing had led to improved marks in all subjects. Jared was pleased to have learned a number of basketball skills, was throwing and catching the ball with much more accuracy, and was participating better in gym class.
- Mrs. Burton reported a decrease in behavior problems and improved competence at most schoolwork but indicated that Jared was still quite isolated socially.
- Mrs. Williams indicated that dressing and morning routines were considerably improved and that Jared was now taking swimming lessons and occasionally played basketball with his sister or with neighbors after school. Jared required strong encouragement to participate in these activities, however, and still showed a preference for passive, isolated activities.

The occupational therapist also observed Jared's actual performance of each of the tasks identified as goals to ensure that they had been achieved as targeted.

Continuing Issues

A decision was made to monitor the social issues to see whether any improvement was observed as Jared became happier at school and more involved in swimming lessons and neighborhood activities. Jared will need to be encouraged to participate in social activities, such as Cub Scouts, drama, or church groups, as appropriate to his interests and his parents' wishes. Jared's family will need to advocate for continued modification at school in subsequent grades and to be aware of some of the issues that may continue to emerge. Keyboarding skills will need to be worked on and Jared may need to be identified as a child with special educational needs in order to ensure that adapted programming is continued. There are no existing parental support groups for parents of children with developmental coordination disorder, so the Williams may need to become affiliated with parent organizations for children with learning disabilities in order to remain informed about advocacy issues within the school system. It is likely that a referral to occupational therapy might again be required if the social skills issues continue to be problematic and also as Jared enters middle school and encounters different teachers for each subject.

➡ Describe the key elements that made this occupational therapy experience successful.

➡ What are the barriers that limit OT from using this approach to treatment planning and implementation? If you have identified barriers, what can you do to remove them?

Occupational therapists in a rehabilitation model see patients, clients, and consumers across the stages of recovery. Each stage of treatment requires a different level of participation with the client (McColl, 1998; McColl, Gerein, & Valentine, 1997). At the biomedical level, the health care team identifies the functional problems of the patient. Treatment is focused on resuming basic self-care and developing support for communication, movement, and occupational performance. At the client-centered level, patients or clients are supported in learning new strategies to successfully perform the activities that are important to them. At the community-based level, rehabilitation aims to equalize opportunities and social integration of people with disabilities. At this level, health professionals work to influence policy, remove barriers, and facilitate participation in work, families, and communities. Independence is the ultimate goal of rehabilitation. At this point, the initiative for control is with the individual, and the rehabilitation program offers ongoing services as problems arise.

Mrs. Bridwell will demonstrate the rehabilitation perspective.

Meet Mrs. Bridwell

Mrs. Bridwell is 63. She is recently widowed and has two grown daughters, ages 32 and 37. She belongs to a Greek orthodox church and is an active volunteer there. Currently, she does not have a significant other, but dates occasionally. Her daughters live in town and visit with their families two to three times a month. She has a close relationship with her sister, who lives about an hour away. She also has a neighbor and several friends who are supportive. Mrs. Bridwell lives in an urban mid-western city in a one-level condominium that is accessible by an elevator from the garage entrance. She has laundry facilities in her home. Prior to her hospitalization, Mrs. Bridwell was responsible for all home management.

Mrs. Bridwell is a retired high school teacher and administrator. Currently, she is an active volunteer at her church and is on the board of directors of the local literacy foundation. She also provides child care for her grandson 2 days a week. Mrs. Bridwell enjoys bridge, golf, travel, reading, and cooking.

Mrs. Bridwell had a cerebrovascular accident (CVA) 3 weeks ago. On the morning of her acute admission, Mrs. Bridwell experienced intermittent numbness in her left upper extremity and noticed that she was slurring her words. Her daughter came by to visit and immediately took her to the emergency room (ER). Upon arrival at the ER, Mrs. Bridwell had significant weakness in the left side of her face and upper extremity, and mild weakness in her lower extremity. The clinical exam, computed tomography (CT), and magnetic resonance imaging (MRI) led to the diagnosis of a right CVA in the middle cerebral artery distribution. Mrs. Bridwell was also found to have elevated blood pressure with resulting atherosclerosis. This was considered to be a primary contributing cause of her stroke. Mrs. Bridwell arrived at the ER 6 hours after the onset of her CVA, so she was not a candidate for TPA—tissue plasminogin activator—a fibrinolytic agent used early on to dissolve thrombi. Her blood pressure was closely monitored and she was provided with supportive care.

Biomedical Rehabilitation

Mrs. Bridwell received occupational therapy, physical therapy, and speech therapy during her 5-day acute hospitalization and her 2-week inpatient rehabilitation stay. She has met the majority of her inpatient rehabilitation goals and has been discharged to home.

She has been referred to home health occupational therapy to address continuing rehabilitation needs in the areas of activities of daily living (ADLs), instrumental activities of daily living (IADLs), and community reentry.

Approach

The person-environment-occupation (PEO) model (Law, Cooper, Strong, Stewart, Rigby, & Letts, 1996) will be used to guide assessment and intervention. Three specific models will influence intervention for Mrs. Bridwell. The rehabilitative approach will use compensatory strategies, environmental modifications, and energy conservation techniques (Dutton, 1995). The Contemporary Task Oriented Approach to Motor Learning (Bass Haugen & Mathiowetz, 1995) is a client-centered intervention centered on personal characteristics and the performance context. Intervention is based on the assumption that a person needs to practice/experiment with various strategies to develop motor skill—an individual as active role in the learning process. Clients are encouraged to use movement patterns that are most functional to them. This model seems to fit well with this client and the home environment intervention setting (Bass Haugen & Mathiowetz, 1995).

A cognitive/behavioral approach will bring neurological deficits that impact behavior into focus. This approach may be used to help the client and her daughters understand limitations that client/mom may be having in terms of executive function and motor functioning. A combination of these three approaches will yield a plan that will support what Mrs. Bridwell wants to do and will involve modifying the environment and preventing secondary conditions.

Identification of Occupational Performance Issues

To establish a rapport and identify, and prioritize occupational performance issues, Mrs. Bridwell was interviewed and the COPM was administered. Mrs. Bridwell was also asked to describe a typical day and week in order to better understand her activity patterns.

Self-Care

- Personal care: During her inpatient rehabilitation stay, Mrs. Bridwell became independent in feeding herself with the use of adaptive equipment. She is able to brush her teeth, comb her hair, and apply make-up with her left upper extremity. She reports some difficulty with managing lids and caps on her toiletries. She is able to dress herself, but avoids pullover shirts because she does not have adequate proximal right upper extremity assisted range of movement. She continues to have difficulty with lower extremity dressing and putting on her shoes with her ankle foot orthosis. Once she is positioned on the tub seat, she is able to bathe herself with the use of a bath mitt and a long-handled sponge. She is independent in toileting and has a bedside commode that she uses at night.
- She expresses an interest in being able to get dressed up in her heels, so that she can go to lunch with her friends. She is also concerned that she has to rely on her daughters to help her get on the tub seat.
- Functional mobility: Mrs. Bridwell ambulates with a quad cane independently in her home. Her daughters provide stand-by assistance for safety outside the home. For long distances, she uses a wheelchair. Mrs. Bridwell is concerned about how quickly she tires when she is walking and is fearful of falling.
- Community management: Prior to her stroke, Mrs. Bridwell drove independently and took care of all of community-based management needs. Currently, she is not driving but hopes to return to this. Her daughter is helping her with paying bills and goes to the grocery store for her every week.

Productivity

- Volunteer work: Mrs. Bridwell is very active in her church. She is chairperson of the annual Fall Festival and is on the liturgy committee. In addition, she is on the board of directors of the local literacy foundation. She attends monthly meetings, is

Table 6-3 Mrs. Bridwell's Occupational Performance Problems (COPM)

Area of Concern	Performance	Satisfaction
Independence in bathing	2	5
Driving	1	1
Providing care for grandson	2	1
Cleaning house	3	3
Going out with friends for lunch/bridge	4	2

involved in grant writing, and recruits volunteers. She reports that she is taking a temporary leave of absence from her duties but hopes to return soon.

- Child care: Mrs. Bridwell provides child care for her 4-year-old grandson 2 days a week. She prepares his meals, takes him on outings, and enjoys playing games with him. She is concerned that she may no longer be able to do this and is worried about her daughter having to make other arrangements.
- Household management: Mrs. Bridwell cared for her home and did all of her cooking prior to the stroke. Currently, she is able to do some light cleaning, such as dusting, but is unable to manage cleaning the bathrooms, vacuuming, etc. Her daughters are preparing her meals for her.

Leisure

Mrs. Bridwell enjoys bridge, golf, travel, reading, cooking, and socializing with her friends. She spends some of her day reading but has difficulty positioning the book. Her friends occasionally drop by, but she is self-conscious about her limited mobility and tires easily. She is not sure when or how she will be able to play golf or travel again.

When asked to indicate the five most important areas of concern, her performance, and satisfaction, Mrs. Bridwell related the information in Table 6-3.

At this point, she has been home for 2 days. Her daughter has been providing the assistance she needs for self-care and IADLs. She has not resumed any of her leisure activities other than reading.

Identify Occupational Performance Components and Environmental Conditions—Person

- Area: Cognitive and sensory system status.
  - ✧ Assessment: Functional Impairment Battery (FIB)
  - ✧ Includes: an assessment of vision (Quintana, 1995), hearing (Schow & Nerbonne, 1982), cognition (Katzman, Brown, Fuld, Peck, Schechter, & Schimmel, 1983), literacy (REALM, Davis, Long, & Jackson, 1993), neglect, language (FAST, Enderby, Wood, & Wade, 1987, Boston Naming Test (BNT) (Morris, Heyman & Mohs, 1989), and depression (GDS, Alden, Austin, & Sturgeon, 1989).
  - ✧ Rationale: The FIB would identify areas that would have significant impact on Mrs. Bridwell's ability to participate in assessments, as well as impact her occupational performance. Understanding concurrent conditions will provide useful insight into selection of appropriate assessments and intervention strategies. If further assessment is needed in the areas of executive function, Kitchen Task Assessment (KTA) would be used (Baum & Edwards, 1993) or Assessment of Motor and Process Skills (AMPS) (Fisher, 1993); if the client requires further assessment of neglect, she would be given full the Rivermead Behavioral Inattention Test (BIT) Battery. If additional concurrent conditions were identified by the FIB, such as low vision, hearing loss, or depression, she would contact the physician to address these needs.
- Area: Awareness of deficits (anosognosia).
  - ✧ Assessment: Informal interview and observation
- Area: Physiological/ neuromotor.
  - ✧ Assessment: Active range of motion, observation, manual muscle tone in right upper extremity, ability to use as a functional assist, endurance, manual muscle strength.
  - ✧ Would not do formal manual muscle test due to decreased tone.
  - ✧ Sensation: Would assess sensation (light touch, pain, temperature, proprioception, and stereognosis).
  - ✧ Balance: Would assess static and dynamic sitting and standing balance by observation.
  - ✧ Rationale: It is important to have a baseline

assessment of all of the above areas. These are components that are typically affected by middle cerebral artery infarctions. All have an impact on occupational performance and the activities that are important to the client.

Strengths of the Client and Therapist

Client Strengths

- Individual—Alert, able to follow three-step directions, memory intact, vision and hearing are within normal limits, has advanced educational degree, does not appear to be depressed, and is able to participate in collaborative process with therapist. Mrs. Bridwell is skilled at organizing church events and problem solving in her board member role with the literacy council and is very personable in general. These qualities may be helpful to her as she organizes and coordinates her support system. She has normal strength in right upper extremity and with near normal return of strength and motor control of left lower extremity. Able to use left upper extremity as a functional assist to brace objects, and left upper extremity is pain free. Static sitting balance is good, dynamic sitting balance and static standing balance are fair.
- Social—Is well liked by her friends and neighbors, who may be willing to provide assistance if needed. Is well connected at her church; church members may be a source of support if needed. May provide assistance with meal preparation, transportation, spiritual support, etc.
- Familial—Daughters live in town and visit frequently; it is likely that they will be an important part of her support network. Her sister lives within a reasonable distance, and they enjoy a close relationship. Daughters and sister may provide assistance with bathing, home management, and transportation.
- Community—Lives in an urban area and has good access to health care and community resources. Mrs. Bridwell will need follow-up medical care and possible occupational performance therapy. She and her family may benefit from attending support groups for persons and families after stroke. Urban area may also offer alternative means of transportation if Mrs. Bridwell cannot return to driving in the near future.

Summarize Mrs. Bridwell's occupational performance strengths:

- Mrs. Bridwell's Strengths
  - Person
  - Environmental
  - Occupational
- Mrs. Bridwell's Limitations
  - Person
  - Environmental

✧ Occupational

➡ What are the factors that could hinder performance?

Therapist Strengths

The therapist has 10 years of experience with persons with stroke across the continuum of care. She is skilled at establishing rapport with her clients and collaborating with them throughout the therapeutic process. She is oriented around an occupational performance model and has gained expertise in standard assessment of stroke. She has been involved in the local support group for persons with stroke and is aware of local resources. She makes a concerted effort to collaborate with other home health team members. In Mrs. Bridwell's case, she will stay in close touch with the nurse about her blood pressure control and with physical therapy concerning her gains in functional mobility. She may also recommend that Mrs. Bridwell and her family meet with a peer counselor to help facilitate her emotional and physical adjustment.

Client's Goals

The therapist and the client will work together to establish goals and outcomes for Mrs. Bridwell. To facilitate this process, the therapist and the client will reflect on the findings of all the assessments. The key areas of concern identified by Mrs. Bridwell via the COPM, the priority activities identified in the Activity Card Sort, and informal interview and discussion will be used as starting points for establishing goals. If Mrs. Bridwell wishes, and it is possible, family will be involved in the discussion. In the event that Mrs. Bridwell identifies many goals, the client will prioritize and select areas that are of immediate concern and establish a starting point for intervention.

Let's look at these factors for each of her goals listed in Table 6-4.

➡ What are the factors that could help Mrs. Bridwell in performing the activities she has identified?

Plan

To ensure a partnership with the client, the occupational therapist would approach the intervention plan by operating under several assumptions identified by McColl, Gerein, and Valentine (1997):

- The client knows what she wants to gain from therapy and what strategies/resources/environmental modifications are best suited for her.
- The client's perspective of her disability and her unique context is the only relevant perspective—she has experience with her disability and her current level of occupational performance, and already has expertise in dealing with many of the issues.
- The occupational therapist serves as a resource, a facilitator, and a supporter by providing information, ideas, and resources following the establishment of rapport and trust.
- How does this approach differ from the traditional medical model? Why might this approach be more useful to ensure long-term outcomes such as quality of life and well-being?

With these assumptions in mind, the occupational therapist would use the goals identified by the client as a basis for discussion—the intervention plan. She might ask the client to identify the three to four most important areas that she would like to focus on initially. The therapist would assist with this process by helping the client consider her options in terms of what is most important to her, and reviewing what tasks and activities are involved to reach a particular goal (e.g., in order to resume social activities, the client needs to be able to get dressed, utilize alternative transportation, etc.).

The client determined that she is primarily interested in:

- Bathing herself independently.
- Getting dressed.
- Resuming playing bridge and reading.
- Identifying alternative means of transportation to her church.

Table 6-4 Mrs. Bridwell's Goals

Goal	*Facilitating Factors*	*Limiting Factors*
Independence in bathing	• Motivated to be independent. • Has adequate executive functioning. • Good strength in right side. • Static sitting balance is good, dynamic is fair and improving. • Bathroom is accessible, has tub bench. • Has support of daughters who will come daily to assist.	• Neglects left side; forgets to wash left extremities; has difficulty locating washcloth and soap if in left visual field. • Weakness in left upper extremity, lower extremity; and dynamic sitting/standing balance affects independence in transfers, safety in bathtub, ability to get soap. • Client is concerned her daughters may not always be available and that she may become a burden. • Daughters not clear on best way to assist/cue client.
Independence in dressing	• Motivated to be independent. • Has adequate executive functioning. • Good strength on right side. • Static sitting balance is good, dynamic is fair and improving. • Independence with upper extremity dressing usually.	• Neglects left side (i.e., has difficulty locating clothing items in left visual field). • Decreased standing balance and right upper extremity active motion limit independent left extremity dressing. • Typically wears skirts and slacks that zip, stockings, and low heels. • Closet/dresser drawer organization limits accessibility.
Increase community mobility	• Motivated to resume active life. • Has good social support network who may be willing to assist with providing transportation. • Lives in urban area with access to alternative transportation.	• Unable to drive at this point due to left neglect, low endurance, inattention, decreased safety awareness. • Is fearful of driving. • Lives in high traffic area.
Continue to provide child care for grandson	• Motivated to spend time with and care for grandson. • Able to interact well with him on a personal level.	• Low endurance, limited functional m mobility, decreased use of left extremities, neglect, and decreased safety. • Daughters concerned about her ability to resume doing this, and client is motivated but not confident.
Increase independence in homemaking	• Motivated to live in own home independently. • Has financial resources to pay outside help. • Able to do light cleaning. • Daughters and friends assisting.	• Low endurance, limited functional mobility, decreased use of left extremities, neglect, and possible decreased safety awareness, especially with hot food prep.
Return to leisure and social activities	• Had many prior activities and interests. • Has maintained contact with friends who are supportive. • Verbalizes interest in reading, bridge.	• Low endurance, limited functional mobility, decreased use to left extremities, neglect, and decreased safety awareness.

Intervention strategies for each area are described:

Bathing

Mrs. Bridwell decided that she would like to sponge bathe at the sink four to five times per week and have her daughters assist her two to three times per week with transferring to the tub seat. She is completely independent in positioning herself for the sponge bath in a chair with arm rests, which she uses to lower and raise herself from the chair. All items needed for sponge bathing are placed in a bucket on the right side of the vanity. Written cues to remember to wash her left extremities were taped to the mirror in her right visual field.

Mrs. Bridwell's daughters were trained in proper body mechanics and tub seat transfer techniques and given information about how to gradually provide less assistance and cues as Mrs. Bridwell progressed (i.e., allow Mrs. Bridwell to perform more of the transfer, phase out verbal cues, etc.). It was recommended to Mrs. Bridwell and her daughters that she dry off while seated on the tub bench as a safety precaution. Soap on a rope was used to limit dropping and retrieval difficulty, and was placed in Mrs. Bridwell's right visual field. A long-handled sponge was selected to assist with washing lower extremities and a hand-held shower was installed. Mrs. Bridwell is encouraged to use her left upper extremity as an assist while bathing.

This sponge bath/tub bench bath schedule allows Mrs. Bridwell more autonomy and helps ease caregiver burden.

Dressing

Mrs. Bridwell initially wanted to focus on organizing her clothing so that she can find what she needs. Mrs. Bridwell elected to have her closet reorganized so that similar pieces of clothing were grouped together. To address her inattention to her left visual field, a bright piece of red tape was placed on the left doorframe of the closet to assist her with scanning all the way to the left. Clothing that was no longer worn was removed from the closet. Drawers were similarly organized and red tape was placed along the upper left inside panel of the drawer.

Since Mrs. Bridwell was independent in upper extremity dressing for the most part, lower extremity dressing was the second focus of intervention. A supportive chair with arm rests was placed near her closet so that she could sit down while putting on her pants, shoes, and socks. Adaptive strategies such as dressing the affected lower extremity first; using a dressing stick, sock aid, and long-handled shoe horn; and wearing elastic waist pants were recommended. Through experimentation with several pairs of supportive shoes and methods, as well as repeated practice, Mrs. Bridwell was able to get her left shoe on with her ankle foot orthosis using a long-handled shoe horn and elastic shoe strings. Mrs. Bridwell is encouraged to use her left upper extremity as an assist while dressing (i.e., draping the clothing article over her left arm). Mrs. Bridwell decided that safe ambulation was more important to her than wearing high heels to church.

Leisure/Social Interests

Mrs. Bridwell realized that she was not ready to resume her weekly bridge game, as it requires high levels of concentration, memory, visual spatial attention, and endurance. She is interested in working toward this goal, however, so alternative card games were suggested, such as spades, war, and solitaire. Adaptive strategies, such as positioning in a supportive chair, using a cardholder, and placing red tape on the left side of the playing table were recommended. Her daughters and close friend were advised of cueing strategies. It was suggested that she play with her grandson as well. As her cognitive abilities and endurance improve, increasingly difficult games could be introduced for longer time periods.

With the support and assistance of her daughter, Mrs. Bridwell might want to consider inviting one or two friends to her condominium for a short visit or lunch. As she gains comfort in social situations and endurance, she may want to consider going to her neighbor's condo or her daughter's home for a small family gathering. Success with these low-demand social events may build her confidence and lead to resuming some of the social activities she enjoys.

Mrs. Bridwell is an avid reader. This is an enjoyable activity for her that does not require much energy. Recommendations for proper positioning of her torso, hips, and left upper extremity in her easy chair were provided. To assist with holding the book, a lap desk and a book holder were tried. Mrs. Bridwell preferred the lap desk, as it was more comfortable and she felt she could use it for other activities. A reading guide was designed to facilitate her scanning to the left margin. Mrs. Bridwell found that reading novels was too frustrating at this point due to her neglect, but she was able to skim through her *National Geographic*, travel magazines, and cookbooks. This seemed to be a good starting point for her.

Alternative Transportation

Mrs. Bridwell agreed that she did not feel ready to resume driving. Alternative means of transportation and destinations most important to her were discussed. Attending church, going to the doctor, and visiting her daughters' homes were priorities at this time. Mrs. Bridwell and the occupational therapist brainstormed possible resources (e.g., family, friends, church members, and community-based transportation systems). Mrs. Bridwell felt that she would be most comfortable with family members and friends assisting with transportation but was concerned about burdening any one person. Mrs.

Bridwell contacted her daughters and three close friends who had expressed willingness to help her. A transportation schedule was devised such that each individual had only one "chauffeuring" responsibility per week. Information about the community-based transportation system was provided. Mrs. Bridwell was informed of the driver's evaluation and training program offered by the local occupational therapy department as a possible future resource.

Context

The intervention occurs within the context of Mrs. Bridwell's home environment and community. The primary goals of home-based occupational therapy are to empower clients to be able to participate in ADLs, home management, care of others, play or leisure activities, and ensure that the outcome is acceptable to clients and their families (Rogers, Holm, & Stone, 1997). This is an ideal place to provide client-centered occupational therapy and to accurately test intervention strategies. In addition, family and involved friends may be more readily available to participate in the process.

Mrs. Bridwell's occupational performance will be optimized in her own familiar environment. She can begin to develop new activity patterns that fit her current abilities, interests, and environment. As she gains cognitive skills, strength, endurance, and functional mobility, the intervention context can be expanded to her community.

Outcomes of Intervention

To determine occupational performance outcomes of the intervention, the COPM was re-administered.

Self-Care

Mrs. Bridwell became independent in sponge bathing at the sink and transfers onto the tub bench with the use of environmental modifications and adaptive strategies. Her daughters continue to be available in the home as a safety precaution while Mrs. Bridwell is in the shower but no longer need to be close at hand.

Mrs. Bridwell is able to retrieve her clothing and get dressed independently with the use of environmental modifications and adaptive strategies. She continues to wear pants with elastic waistbands and supportive shoes. Mrs. Bridwell would like to return to wearing skirts and heels to church in the future. For self-care activities, she has been able to compensate for her left visual neglect.

Mrs. Bridwell has progressed to ambulating with a straight cane and has adequate endurance to move about her home independently. She walks for short distances in the community but continues to use the wheelchair for long distances.

Her alternative transportation system has worked out quite well, although she misses the independence of driving herself. She is interested in pursuing driving in the future.

Productivity

Mrs. Bridwell has not resumed her full duties as chairperson of the church's Fall Festival or liturgy committee but has become involved in a few small projects that she can manage by phone at home. She continues to be on leave of absence from the literacy council board of directors but stays in contact with the group socially.

Her grandson entered a preschool program, so she will not be providing child care for him.

Mrs. Bridwell continues to do some light cleaning and outside help comes in weekly to vacuum, do the laundry, change bed linens, etc. She prepares simple meals for herself and primarily uses the microwave.

Leisure

Mrs. Bridwell is beginning to read short stories and is happy with her progress in this area. She has not been able to resume playing bridge but has hosted a potluck lunch for several of her friends. She reports feeling less self-conscious about her appearance and that she does not tire quite as easily.

Her reassessment of her performance and satisfaction is found in Tables 6-5 and 6-6.

Mrs. Bridwell stated that reviewing her progress helped her to realize the gains she has made.

Continuing Issues/Needs

Mrs. Bridwell continues to have several occupational performance issues. Although she is independent in self-care, she is not able to care for her home independently. She continues to rely on others for transportation and needs assistance with shopping, paying her bills, and heavy cleaning. Her left visual neglect continues to limit her ability to read full-length novels and to play bridge. She feels a bit isolated from her bridge group. She does not feel she is able to travel or play golf like she used to and misses these activities very much. Although she has gained confidence and has adjusted to her new level of abilities, she reports that she does not have the motivation to participate in volunteer work at the level she was prior to her stroke. Although her daughters feel pleased with her progress, they feel increased responsibility for their mother's well-being.

Table 6-5 Mrs. Bridwell's Performance and Satisfaction

Area of Concern	*Performance*	*Satisfaction*
Independence in bathing	8	9
Driving	1	4
Providing care for grandson	1	7
Cleaning house	5	8
Going out with friends for lunch/bridge	5	6

Table 6-6 Mrs. Bridwell's Progress

Occupational Performance Problems	*Performance*		*Satisfaction*	
	Previous	*Current*	*Previous*	*Current*
Independence in bathing				
Driving				
Providing care for grandson				
Cleaning house				
Going out with friends for lunch/bridge				

Note: Revisit the earlier COPM and see what progress has been made.

The rehabilitation process will continue following discharge in several ways. Mrs. Bridwell and her family will be advised of local support groups and peer counselors. Additional options for transportation will be recommended and a referral may be made for a driving evaluation. Alternative volunteer experiences that are less demanding will be explored. An activity-based home program will be designed to promote continued improvement and functional use of her left upper extremity. The occupational therapist will provide her phone number and will place a follow-up call in a few weeks to see how Mrs. Bridwell is doing. If needed, outpatient occupational therapy could be provided.

➧ What are local resources that you can tap to support your clients as they make the transition to independent living?

Barriers and Feasibility

Initial barriers included the sequelae of Mrs. Bridwell's stroke, particularly the left visual neglect, left upper extremity weakness, low endurance, and decreased functional mobility. In addition, Mrs. Bridwell lacked self-confidence and was fearful while walking, during transfers, etc. She had become a widow in the past year and was still adjusting to this major life change. Her daughters were very overwhelmed by their mother's change in health—she had always been active and healthy, and it was difficult to see her requiring so much care. She was also very self-conscious about her appearance in social situations and this impeded resumption of her social activities. By employing an occupational performance perspective, it was possible to overcome many of these barriers through engagement in occupation.

➧ Identify some strategies to help you implement this model within current reimbursement systems.

References

Alden, D., Austin, C., & Sturgeon, R. (1989). A correlation between the geriatric depression scale long and short forms. *J Gerontol, 44*, 124-125.

Bass Haugen, J., & Mathiowetz, J. (1995). Contemporary task-oriented approach. In: C. A. Trombly (Ed.), *Occupational therapy for physical dysfunction* (pp. 510-528). Baltimore: Williams & Wilkins.

Baum, C., & Edwards, D. (1993). Cognitive performance in senile dementia of the Alzheimer's type: The kitchen task assessment. *Am J Occup Ther, 47*(5), 431-436.

Beery, K. E. (1989). *Revised administration, scoring and teaching manual for the Developmental Test of Visual-Motor Integration*. Cleveland, OH: Modern Curriculum Press.

Bruininks, R.H. (1978). *Bruininks-Oseretsky Test of Motor Proficiency*. Circle Pines, MN: American Guidance Service.

Davis, T. C., Long, S. W., & Jackson, R. H. (1993). Rapid estimate of adult literacy in medicine: A shortened screening instrument. *Fam Med, 25*, 391-395.

Dutton, R. (1995). Clinical reasoning in physical disabilities. Baltimore: Williams & Wilkins, 165-174.

Enderby, P. M., Wood, V. A., & Wade, D. T. (1987). Aphasia after stroke: A detailed study of recovery in the first 3 months. *International Rehabilitation Medicine*, 8, 162-165.

Fisher, A. G. (1993). *Assessment of Motor and Process Skills* (Research ed. 7.0). Fort Collins, CO: Department of Occupational Therapy, Colorado State University.

Harter, S. (1985). *The Self-Perception Profile for Children*. Denver, CO: University of Denver.

Katzman, R., Brown, T., Fuld, P., Peck, A., Schechter, R., & Schimmel, H. (1983). Validation of a short orientation-memory-concentration test of cognitive impairment. *Am J Psychiatry, 140*, 734-739.

Law, M., Baptiste, S., Carswell, A., McColl, M. A., Polatajko, H., & Pollock, N. (1994). *Canadian Occupational Performance Measure* (2nd ed.). Ottawa, ON: CAOT Publications ACE.

Law, M., Cooper, B., Strong, S., Stewart, D., Rigby, P., & Letts, L. (1996). The person-environment-occupation model: A transactive approach to occupational performance. *Canadian Journal of Occupational Therapy, 63*(1), 9-23.

McColl, M. A. (1998). What do we need to know to practice occupational therapy in the community? *Am J Occup Ther, 52*(1), 11-18.

McColl, M. A., Gerein, N., & Valentine, F. (1997). Meeting the challenges of disability: Models for enabling function and well being. In C. Christiansen & C. Baum (Eds.), *Occupational therapy: Enabling function and well-being* (pp. 511-512). Thorofare, NJ: SLACK Incorporated.

Morris, J. C., Heyman, A., & Mohs, R. C. (1989). The consortium to establish a registry for Alzheimer's disease (CERAD). Part I. Clinical and neuropsychological assessment of Alzheimer's disease. *Neurology, 39*, 1159-1165.

Quintana, L. A. (1995). Evaluation of perception and cognition. In Trombly, C (Ed.), *Occupational therapy for physical dysfunction* (4th ed., pp. 201-224). Baltimore: Williams & Wilkins.

Rogers, J. C., Holm, M. B., & Stone, R. G. (1997). Evaluation of daily living tasks: The home care advantage. *Am J Occup Ther, 51*(6), 410-422.

Schow, R., & Nerbonne, M. (1982). Communication screening profile: Use with elderly clients. *Ear Hear, 3*(3), 135-143.

Notes

Chapter Seven

Defining the Outcomes of Occupational Therapy Intervention

Mary Law, PhD, OT(c)

Practice Scenario Authors: Mary Ann Bruce, PhD, OTR/L
Nancy Pollock, MSc, OT(c)
Patti LaVesser, PhD, OTR/L

In this chapter, we will examine the issues that influence decisions about the outcomes after occupational therapy intervention. First, let's look at what we mean by outcomes.

An outcome can be defined as the end result, consequence, or effect of an action or actions. For example, a child who has difficulties with attention that affect his social behavior and handwriting may receive occupational therapy services in the school. It is hoped that the results or outcome of the therapy intervention are improved social relationships and handwriting. These outcomes can be documented or assessed using qualitative or quantitative methods.

Levels of Outcomes

In the past, occupational therapists have defined outcomes in terms of occupational performance or performance components. In fact, there was probably more emphasis placed on the assessment and re-evaluation of performance components than the actual tasks and activities that comprise occupational performance. There was an assumption that a change in performance components would automatically lead to change in occupational performance. Research has indicated that these assumptions are not always correct and that an intervention focus on the performance of occupations is more likely to lead to improved outcomes (Trombly, 1995). Trombly (1995) advocates using a "top-down" approach to evaluation and definition of outcome. A "top-down" approach begins with the therapist finding out from the client the specific occupational performance tasks and activities with which he or she is having difficulty.

McColl and Pollock (1998) suggest that assessment in occupational therapy to define outcomes be considered a two-tiered process, consisting of problem identification and problem analysis. In problem identification, therapists facilitate clients to identify occupations that they are having difficulty performing. The results of assessment at this first level (i.e., problem identification) provide the necessary information to define the outcomes of occupational therapy intervention. The second level of assessment, problem analysis, occurs when therapists do further assessment to understand why occupational performance problems are occurring. Information from this level of assessment aids in determining what to focus on during intervention but does not define the ultimate outcome of occupational therapy service.

Issues in Defining Outcomes

What are the important issues to consider when defining the outcomes after occupational therapy intervention? Let's think back to Chapters One and Two. In those chapters, we discussed the importance of focusing on occupation and occupational performance as the core of our practice. The concepts of client-centered practice and how these ideas fit with our beliefs that all persons have the right to make choices about daily occupations were outlined. These ideas lead to specific directions when it comes to defining outcomes in occupational therapy:

- The primary (long-term) outcomes of occupational therapy intervention are occupational performance outcomes.
- The occupational performance issues for intervention, and thus the outcomes, are best defined by the client and/or his or her family or caregiver.
- Secondary (short-term) outcomes, such as changes in performance components or environmental factors, are important only when changes in them lead to changes in occupational performance outcomes.
- The therapist plays an important role in facilitating the client to define the outcomes of therapy through provision of information and enabling them to make choices about occupations that they "want to, need to, or are expected to do" (Law, Baptiste, Carswell, McColl, Polatajko, & Pollock, 1998).

Fearing (1993) has described a method to document occupational performance problems and factors (performance components and environmental conditions) contributing to these problems. She suggests that occupational therapists use a "left side-right side" approach in documenting occupational performance issues. The occupational performance problem is written on the left side with performance components or environmental conditions contributing to the problem written on the right side. An example is provided below:

• Left Side	• Right Side
✧Unable to feed self	✧ Impaired grasp and release
	✧ Lack of adaptive equipment

Let's see how these ideas are applied using practice scenarios. As you read these, think about defining outcomes in a way that begins and ends with occupational performance. We suggest that your learning experience will be enhanced if you work through the questions without moving ahead too quickly to find out what actually happened in each scenario. You can then compare your thoughts to the scenario—there are often many ways to define and measure outcomes.

Meet Peter

Peter is a 34-year-old male who experienced a spinal cord injury while on vacation. He is a family practitioner for a local managed care organization and specializes in working with older adults. He has been happily married for 2 years. His wife is an orthopedic nurse. They do not have children but want to have a child soon. Peter himself is an only child. His father is also a physician and is very well known in the community. Two years ago, when they married, Peter and his wife bought their own home. They currently live in this home, a two-story, single-family residence. There are many young couples moving into their area and renovating the homes in the neighborhood. Peter's hobbies include gardening and some small remodeling tasks around the home.

The spinal cord injury happened when Peter was body surfing. He was rushed immediately to a large hospital where he was given medication to prevent extensive damage to his spinal cord. The injury was at the C5-6 level of the spinal cord. Surgery was performed and Peter was placed in a halo. After leaving intensive care, he returned to a rehabilitation hospital 30 minutes from his home. He was there for 3 months for acute rehabilitation. At the time that this practice scenario begins, he was transferring to outpatient therapy in a hospital about 12 minutes from his home. This transfer was to allow him to return home and minimize the stress on his family for commuting to therapy. He had requested day rehabilitation rather than an outpatient therapy program because he wanted an intense rehabilitation experience. He was also experiencing depression and this daily program was seen as a way to help him manage his depression and build his endurance for return to work.

When the therapist met Peter, he was able to walk but his balance was impaired and he was weak. He had restricted range of motion in his upper extremities, fair minus strength, poor fine motor coordination, and poor endurance. He had bowel and bladder control. He was irritable but thankful that he was alive and not tetraplegic. Peter could get himself dressed but had difficulty with zippers and buttons. He said right away that he was not interested in cooking but would use the microwave. He did not need to cook, as he preferred fresh fruit and vegetables and yogurt, and he and his wife enjoyed going out to dinner.

Occupational Performance Issues

The therapist used a standardized protocol developed locally and an interview to collect information from Peter.

This assessment included brief history (personal and medical); description of previous level of function; identification of client/family goal(s); bilateral upper extremity sensation; strength, range of motion, functional upper extremity assessment; cognition and orientation; balance, coordination, endurance; activities of daily living and instrumental activities of daily living; communication of needs; individual and group skills; activity tolerance; and health habits—use of substances, exercise, etc.

Peter's interests included reading, sports, fitness, medicine, and getting together with friends and family. His primary roles were physician, spouse, friend, and sportsman (running, surfing, swimming, basketball, bicycling). He fears now that he will never be able to father a child. He and his wife are experiencing marital stress due to the traumatic injury and change in their lifestyle. Peter is still wearing a halo brace, is unable to drive, and is beginning to be worried about the family's finances.

- Peter initially identified the following issues:
  - ✧ Unable to write
  - ✧ Unable to efficiently use tools and perform work tasks
  - ✧ Stiffness and tightness in his arms, legs, and back
  - ✧ Muscle spasms in legs and arms
  - ✧ Loss of range of motion
  - ✧ Weakness and decreased strength in arms and legs
  - ✧ Tires easily, depressed mood
  - ✧ Unable to zip and button clothes
  - ✧ Unable to participate at health club
  - ✧ Unable to drive

➠ What are the occupational performance issues identified by Peter?

➠ What other occupational performance issues do you think may emerge over time?

➠ What performance component problems were identified during the assessment process?

Construct a left side—right side diagram (Fearing, 1993) to illustrate the possible relationship between Peter's occupational performance issues and performance components. You can use the notes page at the end of the chapter to do this. We've included one example to get you started (Table 7-1).

Based on your analysis of this information, write down possible short-term and long-term therapy goals for Peter. Also, write down the expected outcome of therapy.

➠ Goal—short-term:

➠ Expected outcome:

➠ Goal—long-term:

Table 7-1 **Left Side—Right Side Diagram**

Occupational Performance Issue	*Performance Component*
• Unable to do zippers or buttons.	• Weakness, lack of fine motor coordination.
•	•
•	•
•	•
•	•

➠ Expected outcome:

Take some time to look at the goals you have described. Are the goals written in occupational performance terms (e.g., improve speed and legibility of handwriting) or in performance component terms (e.g., increase range of motion and strength)? Is there a difference between the short-term and long-term goals in this way? In many instances, the short-term goals may be written to address performance components, assuming that they will affect occupational performance.

Let's take another approach to defining outcomes in this situation. In this case, use Table 7-2 to rewrite Peter's goals. In this instance, we'll link the performance component issues together with the occupational performance issues. We've also added information about measuring the defined outcome. We've provided an example to get you started (See Table 7-2).

Once the outcomes for therapy have been defined clearly, the client and therapist have clear expectations about what will occur through the occupational therapy intervention. Defining outcomes in a clear and measurable way makes it easier for the client and therapist to know when therapy is completed, and reassessment is warranted.

Let's see what actually happened during occupational therapy for Peter.

Peter and his wife met with the outpatient/day rehabilitation team to discuss what aspects of the program he would use. Peter decided to enroll in day rehabilitation in order to increase the time in therapy (6 hours per day, rather than 3 hours per week). He was to see the physical therapist, occupational therapist, and neuropsychologist. Occupational therapy occurred 2 hours per day. The client chose not to participate in the following aspects of the day rehabilitation program: weekly community outing, support group, coping strategies group, cooking group, and the recreation/activity group.

Peter asked to be able to talk about his role of being a physician. His previous treatment environment restricted his interactions with patients and felt he should not share that he was a physician with other patients. We all agreed that he could tell clients he was a physician, but he was not to advise them about their care nor prescribe treatment or make recommendations. Peter agreed that this was the best approach. He also agreed to let us know if clients were asking him to make recommendations. He was kind and caring, well liked by staff, and loved by the other clients.

Peter's goals for therapy were:

1. Strengthen his hands in order to grasp and control objects.
2. Return to work as a physician.
3. Father a child.
4. Return to sports and fitness activities.

The primary focus of occupational therapy intervention was on goals 1, 2, and 4. The occupational therapy program consisted of the following:

Peter was referred to the hand clinic of the rehabilitation department for a thorough evaluation and design of

Table 7-2 Defining Outcomes

Occupational Performance Issue	*Expected Outcome*	*Outcome Measured by*
• Difficulty with handwriting because of weakness, lack of motorcoordination in hands and arms.	• Ability to write at speed and with legibility required for writing prescriptions and medical charts.	• Client self-assessment using the COPM.
•	•	• Standardized handwriting test (using real life situations) measuring legibility and speed.
•	•	•

a treatment program by a certified hand therapist/OTR. This therapist designed a treatment plan in consultation with the client and the day rehabilitation occupational therapist. The program was monitored by the day rehabilitation therapist, who also identified functional tasks for him to do related to the program. Therapy included daily upper extremity stretching to increase range of motion, teaching Peter to complete the range of motion and stretching routine, hand therapy exercise program daily, participating in upper extremity functional activities for occupational performance, and teaching Peter to self-monitor his progress. Peter kept his own record of changes in strength, coordination, and occupational performance.

Peter practiced the fine motor tasks of buttoning his shirt and tying a tie. He practiced writing and tracking the number of words per minute he could write. To do this, a typing book program was used. Peter would copy lines, monitor his time before fatigue, and check for errors. He also practiced writing while interviewing or completing structured forms and using small instruments. The therapist also worked with Peter to develop the transition plan to assist him in participating in work and his fitness center.

The therapist used a client-centered approach during intervention, and this approach enabled Peter and the therapist to develop an excellent working partnership. The therapist facilitated Peter to set his goals, participate in selecting his treatment activities, and to track his progress once the system was identified. The therapist respected his professional role so that he could express it appropriately within the context of his own treatment planning and monitoring, and during daily interactions with clients and therapist. The therapist encouraged him to participate in monitoring his program. He kept records, and the therapist planned the system and met with him daily to monitor his progress and problem solve when new challenges emerged.

The therapist advocated for the client with the team regarding his role and its expression in the program. She took initiative to solicit assistance from an expert when the client's problems were out of her area of expertise. She was honest with the client when he started quizzing her about the anatomy of the hand, suggesting that he should have these discussions with the therapist from the hand clinic. Both therapists were sensitive to the client's occupation and lifestyle.

Outcomes of Intervention

Peter transitioned to 3 days per week in the day rehabilitation program rather than 5 and returned to more independent conditioning in the community and at home. He began to work half-days in a geriatric clinic. He was satisfied with his hand function for work tasks. His efficiency was within acceptable boundaries, but he needed increased time to perform writing tasks. He returned to a modified fitness routine but was unable to maintain this once he returned to work.

Continuing Issues/Needs

Peter continued to experience depression resulting from changes in his performance that kept him from meeting his expectations. He remained concerned about possible inability to father a child. He continued to see the neuropsychologist for these problems.

He returned to work in geriatric medicine 3 days a week, and after 3 months he was full-time. About 1 1/2 years after his discharge, he came by to say hi with a 3-month-old infant in his arms.

Let's turn now to another practice scenario and look at how the outcomes for occupational therapy intervention were defined.

Meet Kyle

Kyle, a 5-year-old boy, began kindergarten in September. He and his 3-year-old sister live with their parents, Gail and Steve Kestle. Gail is a medical secretary and works 3 days per week. Steve is a truck driver and is away from home for long periods of time. Kyle attends school in the mornings and a day care program in the afternoon on the days his mother works.

Kyle has had a history of behavior difficulties. The day care he attended had increasing difficulties managing his behavior. As a result, the family physician referred Kyle to a developmental pediatrician in town, and Kyle was diagnosed as having attention deficit hyperactivity disorder (ADHD) 2 months ago. Although reluctant, Gail and Steve agreed to a trial of methylphenidate. Kyle has experienced some sleep and appetite disturbances, but these are diminishing and they feel there has been a noticeable improvement in Kyle's behavior.

The transition to the school setting has not been easy for Kyle. He has difficulty with the increased structure of the kindergarten program in comparison to the day care program he attends, which is more play-based and allows more freedom. His teacher finds him very impulsive and disruptive to the group, and she is now even more concerned because he has started being physically aggressive with some of the children.

A meeting was held between the teacher, principal, resource specialist, and the Kestles to discuss a plan to deal with the teacher's concerns. Referrals were made for assessment by the school-based occupational therapist, and a request for consultation was made to the district's behavioral consultant.

Occupational Performance Issues

The school-based occupational therapist sees the kindergarten teacher as the client. Kyle's parents are involved in the process but are not the primary target of service. As well, the environment in which the problems seem to be most prevalent is the school, although issues are certainly present in the home.

A phone interview was done with Kyle's mom to inform her of the initiation of service and to get some background information. Kyle's developmental history appears unremarkable. He has always been a very active child, has had difficulty sleeping, has not interacted well with neighborhood children, tends to be rough with his sister, and is very easily frustrated. Kyle's family has always just assumed that this is his personality and was not terribly concerned about his interactions or behavior until his day care staff started to identify it as an issue about 1 year ago. The family also assumed that he would settle down somewhat as he matured.

Mrs. Kestle's main concerns are with Kyle's play and social interaction. She is very concerned that he is being aggressive with other children and worries that he may start to do this at home with his sister. At home, Kyle can be very impulsive and defiant at times, but he is also a very affectionate and loving child. She states that she has a fairly easygoing manner and describes their home as "child friendly and unstructured." Mrs. Kestle is also worried about Kyle's progress at school and wonders whether he may have some kind of learning disability, which is causing him to be so frustrated and disruptive at school.

She and her husband have found Kyle to be somewhat calmer and more focused since he was started on the medication. She feels that he is more willing to follow routines at home and is showing more interest in activities such as building things, doing puzzles, and playing games with the family. Kyle is very active in sports and loves soccer and T-ball, and has recently learned to ride a two-wheeler. He and his father spend a lot of time playing ball together and working on an old car in the garage.

Kyle's teacher, Mrs. Randall, was interviewed using the Canadian Occupational Performance Measure (COPM) and the School Function Assessment (SFA). She identified Kyle's ability to participate in classroom activities, to sustain play activities, to interact positively with classmates, and to follow classroom routines as the areas of top concern. She is also frustrated by the amount of attention that Kyle is demanding from her, which she feels is detrimental to the other children in the class. She has had experience with children with attention problems before but feels that Kyle is more difficult. She is anxious to get some help.

➡ What are the occupational performance issues identified by Kyle's mother?

➡ What are the occupational performance issues identified by Kyle's teacher?

➡ What performance component problems were identified during the assessment process?

➡ What aspects of the environment are important to consider for Kyle and his occupational performance issues?

Construct a left side—right side diagram (Fearing, 1993) to illustrate the possible relationship between Kyle's occupational performance issues, performance components, and environmental conditions (Table 7-3).

Define the outcomes of occupational therapy for Kyle (Table 7-4).

Approach

The occupational therapist examines factors in the child, the environment, the daily occupations, and the interaction between these elements to understand what is happening and to formulate a plan. Developmental theory and neurointegrative approaches are used to frame the assessment process.

The first step is classroom observation. Kyle is not informed that the therapist is there to observe him so that she will likely see typical performance. From the moment he enters the classroom, Kyle is on the go. He drops his coat on the floor rather than hanging it up on the hooks and heads straight for the building center where he begins to stack large plastic blocks. He is redirected to join the other children in the opening exercises in a circle on the floor, which he does after three verbal prompts. He sits with the other children but often keeps some distance from the nearest child. On two occasions, he shouts out an answer when he has not been called on. Prior to the end of circle time, he starts to stomp his feet on the floor repeatedly in an effort to distract other children.

From circle time, the class moves on to a tabletop activity, making a Halloween pumpkin out of construction paper, glue, crayons, and markers. Kyle completes the activity very quickly, does not wait for directions, grabs materials from other children, and then again leaves the table area and returns to the building center. Other children now move on to free time where they can select a center activity. Kyle does not stay for long at the building center once other children join him there and moves from center to center, briefly trying the activities, then moving on. It is difficult to judge his level of skill, as he does not stick with any activities long enough to make a judgment. He does interact with some of his classmates, particularly a few boys, and engages in a bit of roughhouse play until redirected by Mrs. Randall. His interactions are again fairly brief, and he is not observed in any form of cooperative play.

At the recess break, Kyle is observed kicking a ball and running with some other boys. He seems to be very involved and sticking with the outside play. These observations lead to a few hypotheses:

- Kyle has difficulty modulating sensory input.
- Kyle has some learning problems.
- Kyle is delayed in his development and frustrated by the demands in the classroom.
- Kyle is unsure how to behave with his peers and seeks attention inappropriately.
- The classroom is overstimulating to him.

Table 7-3 Left Side—Right Side Diagram

Occupational Performance Issue	Performance Component, Environmental Condition
•	•
•	•
•	•
•	•

Table 7-4 Defining Outcomes

Occupational Performance Issue	Expected Outcome	Outcome Measured by:
•	•	•
•	•	•
•	•	•
•	•	•

- He is used to a very non-directive approach from his parents and is acting out against the teacher's authority.

Further assessment is done on an individual basis. Some standardized tests are used. Although he requires frequent breaks and some redirecting, on a one-to-one basis he is able to complete the tasks expected.

Scores on the Clinical Observations of Motor and Postural Skills (COMPS) and the Peabody Developmental Motor Scales indicate that Kyle is functioning at or above age expectations in motor performance. He did, however, appear to react to tactile input and became upset during the parts of the COMPS that require physical handling. These observations, as well as some behaviors observed in the classroom, suggest that he may have some sensory defensiveness, so the Sensory Profile was completed.

Kyle completed the Developmental Test of Visual Motor Integration and scored in the 38th percentile. He completed the drawings very quickly and made some mistakes due to carelessness; however, there was no evidence of any spatial confusion or fine motor delay that might affect learning to print.

Kyle is developing concepts at an age-appropriate rate in terms of colors, numbers, size, shapes, etc. He can read a few simple words. He can recite the alphabet and print most of the uppercase letters, as well as his name.

Follow-up classroom and playground observations focusing on Kyle's play, using the revised Preschool Playscale, indicate he is not at age level in this area both in terms of social interaction and use of materials.

The classroom environment is likely contributing to his difficulties. It is frequently noisy, very colorful, and somewhat crowded. Children play and work in close proximity to each other. Mrs. Randall has a fairly directive approach and structures the children's time very closely. There is an emphasis on pre-academic learning versus play exploration in her program.

Strengths and Resources

Kyle was very eager to please during the assessment and was able to identify a lot of interests. He says that he enjoys school and looks forward to playing with the other boys at recess. He appears to be following typical development in most areas and has advanced language skills. His parents are very supportive of Kyle and are eager to do whatever they can to help him be successful at school. The district behavior consultant is able to see Kyle next week and will be supporting Mrs. Randall with some ideas for classroom management. Kyle has responded to the trial of methylphenidate and there has been some improvement in his impulsivity and attention.

Client Goals

- Mrs. Randall
  - ✧ Mrs. Randall will recognize the antecedents to Kyle's behavior and intervene before he acts out.
  - ✧ Mrs. Randall will not have to give Kyle more attention than other students in the class receive.
  - ✧ Mrs. Randall will learn some strategies to modify activities to maximize Kyle's participation.
- Kyle
  - ✧ Kyle will participate in classroom activities along with the other children without needing redirection.
  - ✧ Kyle will engage with other children at the building center and cooperate on a project.
  - ✧ Kyle will not show any physical aggression toward other children.
  - ✧ Kyle will continue to enjoy attending school.

Given this information, redefine the outcomes for Kyle. Outcomes will be assessed by completing the COPM with Kyle's mother and teacher.

Plan and Context

The occupational therapist uses both direct and consultative models of service delivery. Kyle is experiencing difficulties in modulating sensory input, particularly auditory and tactile sensation. These difficulties increase his anxiety and cause him to overreact to noise and touch, leading to his aggressive behavior with other children and withdrawal from activities.

The occupational therapist works directly with Kyle in the classroom in regular play activities. This type of intervention in his natural environment is much more likely to generalize to other activities than isolated or withdrawal types of treatment. As Kyle is in a kindergarten class, there are also many naturally occurring opportunities for play-based intervention. The therapist helps Kyle to modulate sensory input and therefore modify sensory stimulation as it occurs in the activity. She uses some calming techniques (e.g., deep pressure touch, joint compression during activities involving different and potentially more stimulating sensory experiences, such as sand or water table play). The therapist also begins to help Kyle recognize both the situations that cause him to become uncomfortable (e.g., close proximity to other children during circle time), and some strategies to avoid those situations, such as having a square of carpet to sit on which defines his physical space more clearly. The therapist and Kyle talk together about a typical day at school, think about or observe times of stress, and then problem-solve together about alternatives. If Kyle is actively involved in this problem solving, he will more likely internalize these strategies.

Once the therapist and Kyle have developed some effective strategies, these are communicated to Mrs. Randall and Kyle's parents so they too can help Kyle to develop alternatives to lashing out at other children and to prepare him to benefit from participation at school. Mrs. Randall also had some good ideas about ways that activities or the classroom environment could be modified to help Kyle and potentially other children as well (e.g., some alterations in the order of activities and a timeout space where children can go to look at books quietly when they feel overwhelmed). Kyle's parents were able to incorporate some calming sensory input into Kyle's daily self-care routine (e.g., wrapping him up tightly in a large bath towel before and after bathing). Once all those involved with Kyle understood the things that set him off, small changes or additions to routines made a significant difference.

Within the classroom there were also some parent volunteers or student helpers. The therapist explained and modeled some strategies to the other personnel as well so that everyone was consistent in their approach and Kyle learned to predict how things went during the day. It was necessary to work with him—role modeling and coaching—in order to help him enter a play group and interact cooperatively. This again is something that others can be trained to do.

In the United States, therapists are typically hired by school boards or school systems to provide this type of intervention. In Canada, therapists may be hired by schools through home care programs or through some children's rehabilitation outreach programs.

Outcomes of Intervention

Kyle was seen twice weekly in class for 6 weeks. After the third week, the occupational therapist had a fairly good understanding of the antecedents to Kyle's behavior and some strategies to deal with them. She met with Mrs. Randall at lunchtime and they brainstormed some ideas together. By this time the behavior consultant had also spent some time in the classroom and developed a behavior program for Kyle. The occupational therapist was aware of the behavioral objectives and also participated in the program.

Kyle's behavior was slow to change, but small, steady gains were seen. His aggression decreased substantially, although his attention was still somewhat inconsistent. He began to initiate social interactions and to play in a more cooperative way with other children at the centers. He moved around less from activity to activity and took more care in his work. He was routinely given positions of responsibility (e.g., handing out materials) and responded very well to these demands. Kyle learned to use the quiet area effectively and to recognize when he needed to go there.

Mrs. Randall reported that she felt more comfortable dealing with Kyle's behavior given her increased understanding of the sensory processing difficulties. She found the ideas and strategies were effective in the classroom and that she was now able to devote equal time to other students. Having classroom assistants who could also monitor Kyle's behavior has eased the load on her.

Mr. and Mrs. Kestle have also found the increased understanding of Kyle's behavior helpful and have made changes in their daily routines that have resulted in a calmer home environment and more cooperation from Kyle. Mrs. Kestle stated that "he is simply easier to live with." He continues to enjoy school and looks forward to going. They are quite pleased with his progress.

Continuing Issues

The occupational therapist will continue to follow Kyle on a consultative basis, available as needs arise. One of the challenges over the next few months will be to prepare Kyle for the transition to grade 1 where the physical environment will be more structured, the expectations for longer periods of independent work higher, and the teacher-pupil ratio lower. The school principal should be involved early on, as the selection of Kyle's teacher for next year will be very important. In addition, his team from this year can start brainstorming what strategies may be effective to pass along for the next teacher.

Barriers and Feasibility

The initial negotiations with Mrs. Randall were somewhat challenging around the intervention planning, because she had a history of working with occupational therapists who withdrew students from the classroom and did direct therapy in another part of the school. This collaborative approach and the presence of the therapist in the classroom were new to her, and initially she was uncomfortable. She did, however, agree to try it. By setting some of the goals from Mrs. Randall's perspective and reinforcing that she was a client as well, the therapist was able to show that this approach could benefit all concerned. The opportunity to brainstorm with the therapists and develop her own ideas about strategies in the classroom helped Mrs. Randall to feel in control and to take some ownership in the process rather than having the therapist make recommendations to her that may or may not have been workable or appropriate from her perspective.

Seeing Kyle intensively (twice weekly) for a shorter period of time was also helpful, as progress was faster and the strategies could be implemented. This therapist has found this more effective than seeing children less frequently over a longer period of time.

The support and cooperation of Kyle's family went a long way toward making this a successful process. The ability of the whole team to be consistent, to communicate effectively, and to work toward similar goals is key.

Meet David

To finish this chapter, we have provided a practice scenario for you to develop on your own. Consider the following practice situation:

David is 41 years old. He lives at home with his mother Alice, who is about to celebrate her 73rd birthday. His father, John, died last year from a heart attack. David has three sisters, two of whom reside close by and one who lives in Vancouver.

David has Down syndrome and a mild heart defect. He attends a local sheltered workshop 3 days a week and a social day program on another weekday. Recently, his mother and sisters have begun to discuss David's future. They are concerned that Alice, who has arthritis, may not be able to continue to care for him at home. They are trying to decide what to do, and they have asked your advice as a community-based occupational therapist.

Following a phone call with Fran, David's eldest sister, and Alice, you gather that they agree that David could cope with a sheltered living situation and would welcome this being set up as soon as possible. Alice stated that her health is not as good as it was even a couple of months ago, and she finds that she does not seem to have the energy to give David as much support as he needs.

Fran takes the phone from Alice and quietly reinforces her mother's concerns, adding that all the sisters are worried about their mother. While Alice says she wants to see David in a comfortable home, she goes back and forth in her willingness to lose him; this has become especially so since John died. Neither parent wanted to see David institutionalized, and Alice's views have not changed, although she appreciates the reality of it all. Alice is also avoiding dealing with details of her estate and is in the process of rewriting her will. Finances are quite solid, according to Fran, but she admits she doesn't know all the details.

➠ What are the occupational performance issues identified by David?

➠ What are the occupational performance issues identified by David's mother?

➠ What are the occupational performance issues identified by David's sisters?

You arrange a visit to their home and, upon arriving at the front door, find David waiting for you. He appears anxious and a little labile. Within only a few moments, he blurts out that he wants to stay with his mother, that he likes his room and does not want to live anywhere else. He does not seem willing to talk about it any further and goes upstairs, shutting himself in his room and turning up his CD player very loud. Nevertheless, you manage to persuade him to sit down and talk with you. You administer the COPM to David, Alice, and Fran separately, clarifying the disparity between their goals.

In essence, the key issues are:

- Reaching a decision about future living accommodations.
- Ensuring David's self-care and social skills are at a level to support residing in a sheltered environment.
- For David and Alice to feel supported during this difficult time in their lives.

Occupational Performance Issues

A lot of very useful information is gleaned from the conversations with David, Fran, and Alice, from which the following issues were distilled:

- Self-care
  - ✧ Independent in dressing, although his mother lays out his clothes for him
  - ✧ Does not travel alone on the bus but can travel independently with a group
  - ✧ Independent in bathing and eating
  - ✧ Able to make his bed and keep his room clean
- Productivity
  - ✧ Attends local sheltered workshop three times weekly; works on assembly line
  - ✧ Helps mother with chores around the house under supervision, takes out garbage, carries groceries
  - ✧ Goes to bingo with Alice; she drives
- Leisure
  - ✧ Goes to day program once weekly for social activities
  - ✧ Occasionally goes to the movies with his sister and her family
  - ✧ Likes to go swimming in the summer
  - ✧ Loves to watch hockey on TV and at the local rink, where he sometimes goes with his brother-in-law and nephew
- Concerns
  - ✧ Has to watch he does not over-exert himself, because of some heart problems
  - ✧ Has some difficulty with coordination
  - ✧ Comprehends most conversations and is able to follow only simple directions
  - ✧ Can read to a grade 1 level and struggles beyond this
  - ✧ Was very sad upon the death of his father and is worried about what will happen to him in the future
  - ✧ Friendly, sociable, and very fond of his nieces and nephew; therefore, very concerned that he will not see them if he has to move away
  - ✧ Only talks with one sister and her husband

➡ What issues related to performance components have an impact on this practice scenario?

➡ What aspects of the environment are important to consider in this practice scenario?

Construct a left side—right side diagram (Fearing, 1993) to illustrate the possible relationship between David's occupational performance issues and performance components and environmental conditions.

Define the potential outcomes of occupational therapy intervention in this scenario.

In Chapter Seven, we have focused on issues related to defining the outcome of occupational therapy. We have described a process that you can use to work through the definition of outcomes and have applied that process using three practice scenarios.

In Chapter Eight, we move on to discuss strategies to ensure that your intervention is occupation-based.

REFERENCES

Fearing, V. G. (1993). Occupational therapists chart a course through the health record. *Canadian Journal of Occupational Therapy*, 60, 232-240.

Law, M., Baptiste, S., Carswell, A., McColl, M., Polatajko, H., & Pollock, N. (1998). *Canadian Occupational Performance Measure* (3rd ed.). Ottawa, ON: CAOT Publications.

McColl, M., & Pollock, N. (1998). Assessment in client-centered occupational therapy. In M. Law (Ed.),. *Client-centred occupational therapy*. Thorofare, NJ: SLACK Incorporated.

Trombly, C. A. (1995). *Occupational therapy for physical dysfunction* (4th ed.). Baltimore: Williams and Wilkins.

RESOURCES

Clinical Observations of Motor and Postural Skills (COMPS). Wilson, B. N., Pollock, N., Kaplan, B. J., & Law, M. (1994). Therapy Skill Builders. San Antonio, TX.

Developmental Test of Visual-Motor Integration. Keith E. Beery (1989). Modern Curriculum Press, a division of Pearson Education. Parsippany, NJ.

Peabody Developmental Motor Scales. Rhona Folio & Rebecca Fewell. (1983). The Riverside Publishing Co., 425 Spring Lake Drive, Itasca, IL 60143.

Preschool Playscale. Knox, S. (1997). Development and current use of the Know Preschool Play Scale. In D. Parham & L. Fazio (Eds.), *Play: A clinical focus in occupational therapy for children*. St. Louis, MO: Mosby-Year Books.

School Function Assessment (SFA). Coster, W., Deeney, T., Haltwanger, J., & Haley, S. (1998). The Psychological Corporation, 555 Academic Court, San Antonio, TX 78204-2498.

The Sensory Profile. Dunn, W. (1999). The Psychological Corporation, 555 Academic Court, San Antonio, TX 78204-2498.

Notes

Notes

Chapter Eight

Doing Occupation-Based Practice

Carolyn M. Baum, PhD, OTR/L, FAOTA

Practice Scenario Authors: Patti LaVesser, PhD, OTR/L
Susan Strong, MSc, OT(c)

The power of occupation has driven the development of our profession since its early leaders recognized that a profession should evolve the conception of a person as an organism that maintains and balances itself in the world of reality and actuality by being in active life and active use (Meyer, 1922). Dr. Meyer set our course when he said the occupational therapist "gives opportunities rather than prescriptions. There must be opportunities to work, to do, to plan, to create, and to learn to use materials." The following practice scenarios illustrate how that vision is operationalized.

Meet Jack

Jack is a 12-year-old boy who has a conduct disorder and attention deficit hyperactivity disorder (ADHD). He has been described as a loner who has difficulty making and keeping friends because of his aggressive behavior. He loses his temper easily, becomes uncontrollably enraged, and often strikes out at anyone nearby. He frequently uses foul language.

Jack is the product of a chaotic home life. By court order, he currently lives with his maternal grandmother and 10-year-old sister because of abuse and neglect by his mother. His mother sees him occasionally, but she has been unable to regain custody because she cannot keep a job on a regular basis and is dealing with alcohol addiction. His father is alive but has not had contact with the family for many years. His grandmother works full-time in the medical records department of a large hospital and has the financial means to modestly support Jack and his sister.

In the first few months after moving in with his grandmother, Jack had several "run-ins" with police over stolen street signs, other vandalism, and two incidents of shoplifting. In each case, restitution was made without Jack having to spend time in juvenile detention. More recently, these types of behaviors have subsided, but Jack continues to stay out past his curfew and then lies about where he has been and with whom. His grandmother suspects him of stealing small amounts of money from her. She has also found cigarettes in his jacket pocket.

School has also been difficult for Jack. In the classroom, he has difficulty paying attention and sitting still. Truancy has been an issue. While Jack's IQ is within normal limits, standardized achievement testing places him 1 to 2 years below age/grade level. He was held back in first grade because of "immaturity" and a suspected learning disability that was never documented. He is presently in the fifth grade and is newly enrolled in a highly structured special education elementary school classroom for children with behavior disorders. Prior to placement in this classroom, Jack has not had an occupational therapy evaluation because his difficulties were not viewed as within the treatment realm of occupational therapy.

Occupational Performance Issues

Jack's teacher, Mrs. Ross, reports that Jack is not doing well in school academically. She states that he does not usually complete homework assignments and has a hard time following school and classroom rules. He appears socially isolated and has few friends, gives up easily during challenging tasks, does not ask for help as needed, and frequently becomes physically aggressive with peers. Still, there are times he does work quietly on his own, and she notes an occasional glimpse of a self-deprecating sense of humor. Overall, she is frustrated, not only with Jack, but also with a classroom of 10 pre-adolescents who are "more difficult to manage" as a group than students she has taught in previous years.

A telephone conversation with his grandmother reveals two sides to Jack's behavior. Although she reports frustration with being frequently unable to manage his behavior, and a particular distaste for his "sassiness" and "cursing," she also describes a young man who looks after his sister and on occasion "goes out of his way to help me around the house." She is very concerned about his behavior in school and his seeming lack of interest in learning. In response to a question you pose about friends, she tells you that she really has not met any of Jack's friends. She feels she cannot allow Jack to bring friends home after school while she is working, and that on weekends she has all she can handle with Jack and his sister.

Approach

Because of his poor school achievement, the inability to complete written work, and problems with peer relations, the school-based interdisciplinary team refers Jack for an occupational therapy assessment to evaluate possible perceptual/cognitive impairments, social/emotional functioning, and self-esteem. Because children with ADHD and/or behavioral problems often have concurrent physical problems as well, a thorough assessment of perceptual and motor skills is necessary to rule out any deficits in these areas.

You decide to use developmental, behavioral, and ecological approaches in your assessment of Jack. To collect information, you will observe Jack in the classroom and on the playground. You will interview Jack, his teacher, and his grandmother. Even though you are a school-based therapist, you know that involvement of Jack's grandmother in any program you develop is essential. In talking with her, you realize she is also in need of help to deal with Jack's behaviors. Both standardized and informal measures will be used.

Some information about Jack was learned from informal discussions with his teacher and grandmother. To supplement this information, you decide to interview Jack's teacher, his grandmother, and Jack using the Canadian Occupational Performance Measure (COPM) (Law, Baptiste, Carswell, McColl, Polatajko, & Pollock, 1998).

- Mrs. Ross identifies Jack's inability to attend to classroom instruction, to complete his work, and to interact appropriately with other students as her main concerns.
- Jack's grandmother describes similar priorities at school and with peers, but would also like to improve Jack's compliance with rules at home and decrease his use of profanity.
- During the interview with Jack, he has difficulty identifying any problem areas for himself, so you use the time to gather information about his family, friends, self-care, school, and leisure interests. When asked how he feels about school this year, Jack replies that he "hates school" and "feels like he is in prison." He reports that his grades this year are "not so good." He describes one friend, a boy who is much younger, but adds that he generally eats lunch and plays alone. The two most difficult things about school are "most of the kids are dumb" and "the teacher picks on me." The best thing about school is "nothing." He reports enjoying computers, drawing, and listening to music. He is glad he is living with his grandmother. He states that "maybe" he would like to do better for her sake.

To formally assess Jack's perceptual and motor skill development, the Test of Visual-Perceptual Skills (TVPS), the Test of Visual-Motor Skills (TVMS), and the Bruininks-Oseretsky Test of Motor Proficiency-Screening are administered. Jack is compliant but fairly quiet during this process. He makes little eye contact with the therapist. He does not engage in conversation, except to make an occasional self-disparaging remark. His attention span appears short and he requires frequent redirection to the task. After about 40 minutes of testing, Jack announces that he is done. With coaxing, he is able to finish the last few items on the Bruininks. He is allowed to return to his classroom where he punches another student on the arm who is standing near the classroom doorway. He appears angry and near tears as the teacher gives him a time out. You return to your testing room, score his tests, and find that his performance is above average in all areas.

The second assessment session begins with Jack filling out the Tennessee Self-Concept Scale (TSCS). His reading skills seem adequate, although he asks for clarification of a statement at various times. He completes it and hands it back to you without any further questions. Next, Jack is asked to choose an activity. After much deliberation and stating he has no interest in anything, Jack chooses to decorate a baseball type cap with fabric paints. This activity allows you to observe his ability to make a choice, follow directions, complete a task, problem solve, appropriately use materials, and attend to the task. Despite his initial procrastination in beginning the activity, Jack is able to follow written directions well and appears to respond to verbal praise for his efforts. About halfway through the project, Jack needs to be prompted to continue the activity to completion. He frequently criticizes his own work and abilities as he proceeds, and when the cap is finished, he decides it looks stupid and refuses to try it on or to take it with him back to class.

Jack's total score (33) on the TSCS indicates a low self-concept. This can be interpreted as him feeling doubtful about his own self-worth. Subscale scores also reflect that he avoids taking responsibility, has difficulty expressing himself, and is oppositional.

During one final assessment session, Jack is paired with another 12-year-old, David, to evaluate social skills. The two boys are given the directions to work together to "choose an activity." After nearly getting into a fight over what to choose, Jack takes over by announcing that they will play Monopoly. It is clear that Jack is used to getting his way, and David sulks but gives in. When they sit down to play, Jack chooses the game piece he wants and gives David and the therapist their choice of what is remaining. Jack is bossy and controlling throughout the playing time and rather than land on an "undesirable" space, often cheats. David clearly is not enjoying the interaction with Jack and "quits" periodically. When time is up before the game is over, Jack declares he is the winner because he has the most money. He continues to taunt David, calling him a "loser." The therapist quickly moves in to prevent a fight from breaking out.

Jack has a normal IQ and no apparent deficits in perceptual and motor abilities. He responds to positive reinforcement. Jack has a variety of leisure interests and abilities, including art, music, and working on the computer. His grandmother is supportive and wants to work with him to do better. He has a good relationship with his sister. His classroom teacher is supportive.

Summarize the assessment findings below:

- Jack's Strengths
  - Person
  - Environmental
  - Occupational
- Jack's Limitations
  - Person
  - Environmental
  - Occupational

These assessments and observations lead to the following hypotheses:

- Jack's inability to succeed academically does not appear to be due to any cognitive, perceptual, or motor deficit, but rather to his short attention span, impulsiveness, and maladaptive strategies to problem solve.
- Jack is unable to interact appropriately with peers due to immature and poorly developed social skills, along with poor self-concept. He lacks skills in cooperating, compromising, and communicating his opinions effectively. He copes by becoming angry or bullying others.

After more discussion with Jack, these goals are set:

1. Do better in school.
2. Control his behavior and learn to ask for help.
3. Make some friends.
4. Get along better with his grandmother.

The therapist develops long-term goals and short-term goals to meet the goals that Jack has set.

- Long-term: Develop strategies to improve school achievement that address increased attending skills, decreased impulsiveness, increased participation in class, and increased ability to follow classroom rules.
- Short-term: Jack will identify his feeling of frustration before he becomes overwhelmed and/or tunes out, and will appropriately ask a teacher for help or permission to take a 2-minute break with 75% success.
- Long-term: Improve peer relations through developing skills to recognize problem situations, problem-solving strategies to deal with these situations, and improve social communication.
- Short-term: Given a supportive small group and verbal cueing as needed, Jack and two peers will successfully negotiate to choose a therapeutic activity on three of five consecutive sessions.
- Long-term: Improve behavior at home through increasing rule compliance and decreasing use of profanity.
- Short-term: With input from the occupational therapist and social worker, Jack's grandmother will develop behavior management skills so that an age-appropriate curfew is established. Jack follows guidelines for letting his grandmother know where he is going and when he will be home, and Jack communicates who he will be with 90% of the time.

➠ What were the occupation-based strategies that the therapist used for assessment with Jack?

✧ What occupations are meaningful to Jack?

✧ How would you find out this information?

Plan and Context

➠ Think about and list your ideas for occupation-based intervention with Jack.

Let's see what happened:

Both direct and consultative models of service delivery will be used by the occupational therapist.

Social skills goals related to problems with peer relations will be addressed through a small, activity-based group. The group will have two to three participants working with the occupational therapist. This will allow students to develop a relationship with an adult while simultaneously learning ways of interacting productively with peers. The focus of the small group activities will be on cooperation, sharing, showing respect for each other, initiating and responding to conversation, developing self-awareness, labeling emotions, and giving/receiving corrective feedback. Developmentally appropriate games, academic tasks, and hypothetical stories will be used, along with actual social activities that would naturally occur in a school setting. Members of the group will practice skills that are first modeled by the therapist. Verbal and physical prompts will be used to develop Jack's problem-solving strategies. Appropriate responses will be positively reinforced. These strategies, based on behavioral and social learning approaches, may be effective with Jack because there is evidence in the literature to suggest that children with a conduct disorder often exhibit a learning style through which they are motivated to seek reward and to avoid punishment. Positive reinforcement of appropriate behaviors will also serve to enhance low self-concept. It has been shown that children with poorly developed social skills require highly structured programs that emphasize learning and practice of life skills in context. Several activities seem to work well with Jack, including games that require appropriate social responses.

Consultation is provided to Mrs. Ross, the classroom teacher. Since she is feeling overwhelmed by her class in general, the occupational therapist helps her to identify the leaders in the class and the behaviors they exhibit that contribute to the disruption. She then helps the teacher to develop programs to channel their behavior in more appropriate ways. Specifically related to Jack, the occupational therapist and teacher together use a behavioral approach to better understand Jack's problem and needs, to generate ideas for solutions to the problems, and to strategically plan intervention. One idea is that of the classroom teacher developing a behavior contract with Jack.

The occupational therapist also works with the school social worker in this case to develop a behavior management program for home. Jack's grandmother is very willing to receive training.

Jack is seen two times per week outside of class time in the small groups setting as described above. The occupational therapist also visits the classroom for short periods of time at least twice a week to see how the behavior contract is going and to check on the overall performance of the class. She meets with Mrs. Ross one time per week when they review the performance and progress of Jack and each of the different children in Mrs. Ross's classroom who are also receiving occupational therapy services.

Jack is working with the tai chi coach at the local YMCA to work on endurance and have an appropriate outlet for his temper. He is beginning to make a few friends at the YMCA.

Outcomes of Intervention

Over the course of the first semester, Jack's progress is slow but steady. He seems to enjoy coming to the occupational therapy small groups sessions. Although his willingness to talk in the group setting was minimal at first, he seems to be developing an interest in interacting with one of the other two members, a boy who is fairly outgoing but who has similar issues of attention and impulsivity.

In the classroom, Mrs. Ross reports that the class as a whole is better behaved now that she has channeled some of the previously noted acting-out behaviors into more appropriate activities. She sees that Jack is making attempts to complete some of his assigned work, particularly when she breaks his assignments down into small, more manageable units. Jack's angry outbursts still occur but with less frequency. For the second semester, the occupational therapist decides she can cut back on classroom participation and possibly expand the number of students seen in the group to five to six (a classroom aide will assist her so that the staff to student ratio remains small). The "club" will focus more on social activities, planning and carrying out several community outings, as well as participating in and carrying out plans for a spring dance at school.

At home, his grandmother reports that he has stopped leaving the house at night without her permission and is more communicative about where he is going and who he is with. Still, Jack continues to have times where he loses his temper, is disrespectful, and uses profanity. His grandmother credits the behavior management program with some of the progress and feels his increased engagement in school activities is also effective. She continues to worry about his lack of friendships outside of school and that he will get back in with "the wrong crowd."

Continuing Issues/Needs

As Jack continues on to the middle school years, prevocational interests and future vocational potential will need to be addressed. As an occupational therapist on the interdisciplinary team, you would also want to be monitoring Jack's situation so that the appropriate recommendation for placement could be made for the following school year—possibly a move back to a regular classroom, full-inclusion setting.

Jack's mother continues to drift into and out of his life, and recently she has expressed an interest in regaining custody of her two children. There is a possibility that she will move in with her mother and her two children in the near future. If that takes place, it will be necessary to train her in the same behavioral techniques currently being employed by the grandmother. It will also be very necessary to monitor Jack at this time, as transitions are difficult for him.

The issue of peer relations outside of school should also be addressed. This could possibly be accomplished by getting Jack involved in some type of age-appropriate organized sports team, club, or Scouts. He would be asked to describe his interest in any of these activities so that an appropriate match might be identified. Another option may be to involve him in a program such as the Big Brothers of America, in which a male adult (often a college student) would provide him with companionship and serve as a positive male role model and mentor.

Barriers and Feasibility

The prognosis for conduct disorder is not good—often these children or adolescents will go on to have life-long difficulties, including adult personality disorders. The rate of high school dropouts among this population is high. At any rate, progress in changing established behaviors is often slow.

Jack's grandmother is aging, and there is no guarantee how stable a home life he will have given the current situation with his mother. The presence of a male role model in his life may be difficult to achieve.

Successful experiences in relationships, learning, and vocational skills should be organized to support him and prepare him with the skills for life.

➡ What occupation-based strategies can be put into place on a long-term basis to support Jack's continuing functioning?

➡ What community resources can help the grandmother, the mother, and Jack to continue making progress?

➡ What could occupational therapists do to improve the availability of services to work with children and youth with ADHD?

Meet Michael

Michael, a 24-year-old student, moved to a large city to go to college. He began to experience paranoid thoughts. After completing one computer course, he had auditory hallucinations and left school. He spent the remainder of the school term writing in a journal about spirits and science without his family's knowledge. Student health services linked him with a psychiatrist. He was prescribed psychotropic medications that reduced Michael's paranoia. Michael returned home to live with his parents with psychiatric follow-up at a community psychiatric clinic.

Michael is a first generation Canadian of Polish decent. His family has a history of working hard and sacrificing to establish a family business and to ensure that Michael, the oldest son of four children, has a good education and an easier life than his parents did.

Michael indicated he wanted to work. His psychiatrist referred him to occupational therapy to provide information about Michael's work interests, skills, and suitable work environment; to assist with developing a rehabilitation plan; and to help Michael develop his self-confidence.

Table 8-1 Michael's Role Checklist

Past Roles	*Present Roles*	*Future Roles*
Student		Student
Worker		Worker
Volunteer		
Home maintainer	Home maintainer	Home maintainer
Friend		Friend
Religious participant	Religious participant	Religious participant
Hobbyist		Hobbyist

Occupational Performance Issues

The occupational therapist met with Michael and began by gathering historical occupational information through interviews. Michael spoke of being a rather nervous, anxious student in grade school, who was socially isolated and did not participate in any extracurricular activities. He had average grades and particularly enjoyed reading and woodworking. His work history includes working one summer as a gas station attendant. Throughout high school, he worked on and off at the family hydraulics business grinding, drilling, tapping holes, and sweeping. He reported enjoying working with his hands but felt he was "letting his family down" by his work performance not being at competitive standards. Also, he felt uncomfortable around one of the other employees. He had enrolled in computer courses because it was so different than working on a shop floor with his father. He was seen as having many future work opportunities and was acceptable to his family.

Together, Michael and the occupational therapist completed and discussed the Role Checklist (Oakley, 1985) to examine past, present, and future occupational roles (Table 8-1).

His present role involvement represents a decrease compared to his past role involvement. He valued student and worker roles, with more emphasis on worker, seeing student as a means to obtain work. He did not view volunteer or caregiver roles as valuable at the time. He currently spent his days doing household chores, attending Mass, and sleeping.

The therapist used the Canadian Occupational Performance Measure (COPM) to summarize issues, and name and prioritize occupational performance problems from Michael's perspective.

1. Michael wants to work "at a regular job" but sees difficulties concerning:
   - The quality of his work due to anxiety and dealing with auditory hallucinations when working ("people say things about me")
   - Stamina to work full days
   - Dealing with supervisors and co-workers
2. He desires friends but lacks experience and confidence, and fears repercussions once someone knows he has a mental illness.
3. He is not satisfied with his weight gain and lack of participation in leisure activities that were once a part of his life.

Michael is a courteous, personable individual who is clean and appropriately dressed. He has a strong desire to work. He sees work as "being more productive... having something to look forward to when I get up." "I enjoy working. It keeps me going and I do not think about my problems." Pursuit of work is supported by his family's work ethic; his work experience and work habits developed at the family business. His mental illness is stable but he must still manage dealing with auditory hallucinations from time to time. He is aware of his illness and the need to manage it. The therapist has a strong desire in helping Michael achieve his goals and a belief in Michael's abilities to bring about change.

At this time he is comfortable with living at home, performing household chores, and his ability to care for himself. The most important occupational performance problems and ratings by Michael are listed in Table 8-2.

Approach

By using the Person-Environment-Occupation Model (Law, Cooper, Strong, Stewart, Rigby, & Letts, 1996), the therapist is able to analyze occupational performance problems and conceptualize interventions to improve person-environment-occupation relations.

A psycho-emotional approach is selected to use cognitive-behavioral assessments and interventions to deal with the anxiety, auditory hallucinations, and lack of self-confidence that contribute to the four occupational performance problems.

Table 8-2 Michael's Occupational Performance Problems		
Occupational Performance Problems	*Performance*	*Satisfaction*
Obtaining and maintaining a job	3	2
Making friends	1	1
Obtaining and maintaining a comfortable weight	6	2
Participating in leisure activities	6	2

Using a socio-adaptive approach, the therapist, with Michael, is able to explore, understand, and adapt to his family's culture and society's responses to persons with mental illness. An environmental approach facilitates the therapist to explore what environmental conditions enable Michael to optimally learn and perform at work, socially, and in leisure activities.

- Michael's Strengths
  - Person
  - Environmental
  - Occupational

- Michael's Limitations
  - Person
  - Environmental
  - Occupational

Michael and the therapist both have strengths and resources that they bring together to address the occupational performance problems. The therapist brings knowledge of vocational and avocational resources and experience at facilitating clients, such as Michael, to reach their occupational goals.

➠ What occupation-based strategies would you use to help Michael with the occupational performance issues he has identified?

Michael's Goals and Plan

- Perform work activities while managing anxiety and hallucinations.
  - ✧ Work part-time in a consumer-driven affirmative business while practicing cognitive-behavioral coping techniques
  - ✧ Maintain a work journal about confidence, performance ratings, and comments
- Identify types of work and work environments that match Michael's interests and abilities.
  - ✧ In 6 months time, participate part-time in a comprehensive vocational assessment/work trial for 2 months
  - ✧ Complete the Work Environment Impact Scale (Moore-Corner, Kielhofner & Olson, 1998) and Worker Role Interview (Velozo, Kielhofner, Gern, Lin, Azjar, Lai, & Fisher, 1999) after the work trial and experiencing the affirmative business to identify person-environment barriers and supports
- Regain participation in previous leisure activities.
  - ✧ Operate electronic remote control airplanes on a weekly basis
  - ✧ Join a local model airplane club in 3 months time
  - ✧ Join the local library and take out books; read a book per month
- Lose 25 pounds.
  - ✧ Discuss with mother the wish to lose weight and request low calorie meals/snacks
  - ✧ When weather permits, ride bicycle or walk each day
  - ✧ Record weight weekly and participate in exercise activities
- Be comfortable socializing over a cup of coffee.
  - ✧ Visit coffee shops on own and document comfort level and which shops have a more comfortable environment
  - ✧ Socialize with someone from the affirmative business over coffee by 6 months
  - ✧ Socialize with someone from the model airplane club over coffee by 9 months

Context

An affirmative business was selected as a safe, accepting environment to begin testing ways of managing his illness while working. The business offers a community of consumers who act as role models and share strategies for coping with the daily battle with mental illness. The setting is flexible to individuals' needs. The type of work at the affirmative business has value to Michael (environmental recycling, disassembling parts) and will be conducive to success because he is using skills from previous work experience on a part-time basis.

Operating airplanes was the past leisure activity that Michael was most interested in pursuing and now fits his older life stage. He felt most confident of his knowledge and performance in this hobby to provide the basis for joining a club. A club was chosen as a next step to gaining social experience. Socialization surrounds an enjoyable activity and would be a less anxiety-inducing context.

Michael needed to engage his mother's support to make it possible to lose weight.

Plans to socialize over coffee involved selecting a place with an environment that was the most comfortable to Michael and gradually increasing demands. Affirmative business participants were accepting of Michael's circumstances, whereas coffee with a club member required Michael to answer difficult questions. In preparation, Michael previously role-played with the therapist, practicing potential answers to questions together with cognitive statements that he could tell himself to manage the situation.

➠ What did the occupational therapist do in this situation to ensure that intervention was occupation-based?

Table 8-3 Michael's Performance and Satisfaction

Occupational Performance Problems	*Performance*	*Satisfaction*
Obtaining and maintaining a job	5	4
Making friends	5	5
Obtaining and maintaining a comfortable weight	5	4
Participating in leisure activities	8	8

Outcomes of Intervention

Every 2 months, interventions were evaluated by examining the extent to which objectives were met (Table 8-3). The following outcomes were reviewed with Michael:

1. Changes in work journal entries concerning confidence and performance ratings and general comments.
2. Identification of suitable types of work and work environments, and barriers to employment.
3. Participation in leisure activities: model airplanes club, reading.
4. Changes in record of weight and exercise.
5. Experiences with socializing and levels of comfort.

At 9 months, after the original plan had been implemented, the original occupational performance problem areas were re-rated using the COPM with the results listed in Table 8-3.

Michael was pleased with his performance at the affirmative business and recognized gains in his ability to compartmentalize the auditory hallucinations. His self-confidence had increased and he was managing his anxiety to his satisfaction within the particular context. When asked to rate his performance and satisfaction in obtaining and maintaining a job, he gave increased but only moderate ratings, commenting that the work was not at the level of a "regular job" (i.e., less hours, slower pace, accepted his illness), and he had difficulties with multiple-step, new tasks. He acknowledged that the goals regarding socialization had been met, but now his expectations of himself had increased. He found that losing weight was harder than he had expected and the goal of 25 pounds had not been reached. He was enjoying the airplane club and was satisfied with his participation.

Revisit the earlier COPM and see what progress has been made (Table 8-4).

Continuing Issues/Needs

Michael increased his hours at the affirmative business and set new goals for himself regarding work pace and quality. He was linked with a job club where members wrote résumés, shared job-finding strategies, and role-played job interviews. A staff member also provided support, facilitated discussions, and identified resources as required. Michael was a rather quiet member, and initially his anxiety was high. He took out a membership at the YMCA to exercise, lose weight, and socialize.

Since additional supports and resources were in place, the occupational therapist reduced the frequency of meeting with Michael to once every 3 months to monitor his changing needs.

Barriers and Feasibility

Michael continued to deal with others' attitudes toward mental illness and anxiety in social situations. He was able to successfully enter and participate in the vocational assessment, affirmative business, and job club in part because these environments were (or became, with the therapist's intervention) flexible to his needs and accepting of his mental illness. "Regular work" tends to not be as flexible or as accepting. Michael would need to find a niche where he could contribute on a part-time basis and where staff was flexible in exchange for appreciating his other qualities. Key to success was supporting Michael's determination and willingness to be an active agent in his recovery process. He needed to experience challenges and successes in meaningful occupations while perceiving a measure of control. His interests, values, skills, and abilities matched the occupation requirements and environmental demands. In sum, the quality of the fit between Michael, his occupations, and environments is essential for success.

Table 8-4 Michael's Progress

Occupational Performance Problems	*Performance*		*Satisfaction*	
	Previous	*Current*	*Previous*	*Current*
Obtaining and maintaining a job				
Making friends				
Obtaining and maintaining a comfortable weight				
Participating in leisure activities				

➠ What are local resources that you can tap to support your clients as they make the transition to work and independent living?

References

Law, M., Baptiste, S., Carswell, A., McColl, M., Polatajko, H., & Pollock, N. (1998). *Canadian Occupational Performance Measure* (3rd ed.). Ottawa, ON: CAOT Publications.

Law, M., Cooper, B., Strong, S., Stewart, D., Rigby, P., & Letts, L. (1996). The person-environment-occupation model: A transactive approach to occupational performance. *Canadian Journal of Occupational Therapy*, 63(1), 9-23.

Meyer, A. (1922). The philosophy of occupation therapy. *Archives of Occupational Therapy*, *1*, 1-10.

Oakley, F. (1985). The Role Checklist. Occupational Therapy Services. Department of Rehabilitation Medicine, Clinical Center, National Institutes of Health. Washington D.C.: U.S. Government Printing Office, 526-620.

Moore-Corner, R. A., Kielhofner, G., & Olsen, L. (1998). *Work Environment Impact Scale*. Chicago, IL: Model of Human Occupation. Chicago Clearinghouse, University of Illinois at Chicago.

Velozo, C., Kielhofner, G., Gern, A., Lin, F .L., Azjar, F., Lai, J. S., Fisher, G. (1990). Worker role interview: toward validation of a psychosocial work-related measure. *Journal of Occupational Rehabilitation*, 9(3), 153-168.

Resources

Bruininks-Oseretsky Test of Motor Proficiency-Screening. Bruininks, R. H. (1978). American Guidance Service, 4201 Woodland Road, Circle Pines, MN 55014-1796.

Oakley, F. (1985). The Role Checklist. Occupational Therapy Services. Department of Rehabilitation Medicine, Clinical Center, National Institutes of Health. Washington D.C.: U.S. Government Printing Office, 526-620.

Tennessee Self-Concept Scale (2nd ed.).William Howard, Fitts & W. L., Warren, (1996). Psychological Assessment Resources, Inc., 16204 North Florida Ave., Lutz, FL 33549.

Test of Visual-Motor Skills, Revised (TVMS-R): Morrison F. Gardner, (1995). Psychological and Educational Publications, Inc., P.O. Box 520, Hydesville, CA 95547.

Test of Visual-Perceptual Skills (non-motor) Revised (TVPS): Morrison F. Gardner, (1996), Psychological and Educational Publications, Inc., P. O. Box 520, Hydesville, CA 95547.

Notes

Section Four

Making Occupation-Based Practice Happen

This section is designed to bring all of the ideas in the workbook together and to explore a model that can be used for implementing a client-centered, occupation-based practice. The Occupational Performance Process Model helps therapists ensure that a partnership with a client is developed from the very beginning of the therapy encounter. We again use case scenarios to assist you with learning this process.

Chapter Nine

Occupation-Based Practice: Putting It All Together (Part One)

Sue Baptiste, MHSc, OT(c)

Practice Scenario Authors: Cynthia R. Ballentine, MSOT, OTR/L
Debra Stewart, MSc, OT(c)

In this chapter, we will begin to explore the Occupational Performance Process Model (Fearing, Law, & Clark, 1997), a model which was developed as a method to ensure that client-centered principles and the person-environment-occupation relationship is at the core of occupational therapy practice (Figure 9-1).

Occupation Performance Process Model

As you can see, the model has seven stages working in a clockwise direction. In Chapter Nine, you will become familiar with stages 1 through 4; in the following chapter, Chapter Ten, you will work more closely with stages 5 through 7. So, let's get started and see how this process can help you increase your comfort with working in a client-centered, occupation-based manner.

Stage 1: Name, Validate, and Prioritize Occupational Performance Issues (Screening)

As the initial step, this stage helps to screen service needs from the viewpoint of the client. Since not every issue or problem will require input from an occupational therapist, this is a good time to identify any other assistance that the client may define as important and/or helpful. This is a very critical stage during which the underpinnings for the ongoing relationship are laid. Thus, it is vital that as the therapist, you spend time to develop this relationship as a true partnership, applying the key behaviors of a client-centered therapist (CAOT, 1997):

- Listening to what the client understands, values, and chooses.
- Helping the client see what might be possible.
- Respecting the client's abilities to cope.
- Facilitating the identification of needs.
- Providing information.
- Emphasizing open and honest communication.
- Not overwhelming the client with bureaucracy.

Naming occupational performance issues can be approached by gathering information from a variety of sources if the client is a group or organization. If the client is an individual, then the use of the Canadian Occupational Performance Measure (COPM) (Law, Baptiste, Carswell, McColl, Polatajko, & Pollock, 1998) is an excellent method for defining specific issues that are of central importance to the client. Clients may define occupational performance issues that are key now or may prove to be important for them later. There is potential for a dilemma to develop when the client and the therapist disagree regarding the importance of specific issues; however, this is where attendance by you, the therapist, to the core philosophy of client-centered practice is essential. Thus, problems and differences of opinion can be minimized, though not removed entirely.

Reinforcing the validity of each defined occupational performance issue with the client is also an essential piece of the puzzle. This allows for priorities to be set and the beginning of a plan for the partnership to unfold.

Stage 2: Select Theoretical Approach(es)

While many clinicians in occupational therapy may tend to shrug off the value of defining theory associated with day-to-day practice and may appear perturbed when asked what theoretical approaches they apply to their practice, this is an essential element of sound practice and one which we should strive to bring into our realm of conscious decision-making.

The word *approach* has been used in stage 2, since it provides a broad enough opportunity to include models, theories, frameworks, and paradigms. The last thing we need to worry about here is the semantic arguments concerning these terms in general! So, let's assume that any of such words or terms can be applied to this stage. In this era of rapid change and challenge in health care, it is critical that we engage personally in the search for defining practice based on evidence, and therefore there is undoubtedly pressure to use proven theories or methods in our practice; if we base our practice on a well-reasoned basis of theory, we are practicing in an autonomous, responsible, and responsive manner.

Such theoretical underpinnings can be specific or generic. In defining your practice overall, you may find that you generally ascribe to certain theories or models that define the person-environment-occupation relationship; however, when defining specific directions for certain clients, you may elect to base your plan on very precise models that apply in a certain case. It is very important to realize that changes in theoretical baselines can occur frequently during the course of a therapeutic partnership. You should not feel constrained by what you identified in the beginning.

Stage 3: Identify Occupational Performance Components and Environmental Conditions

At this point in the cycle, you need to think about what occupational performance components and environmental conditions are impacting (or may impact later) on how the client can achieve his or her occupational performance goals. It is most important to ensure that the

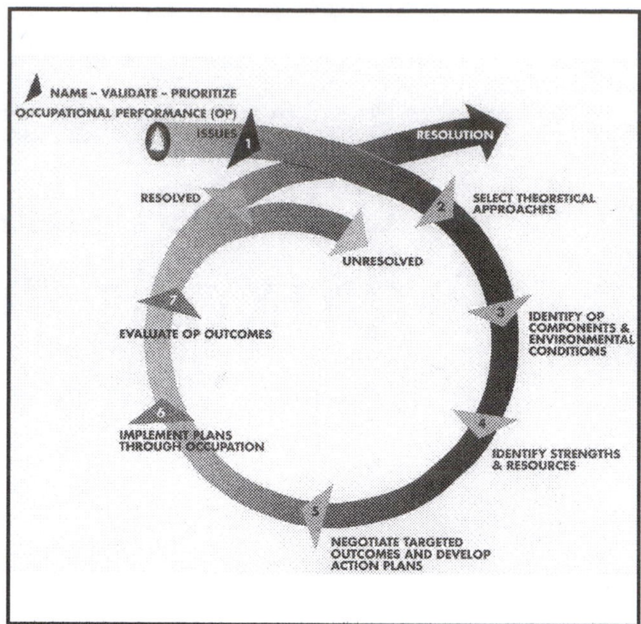

Figure 9-1. Occupational Performance Process Model (adapted from Fearing et al. (1997). *Canadian Journal of Occupational Therapy, 64,* 11, and reproduced with permission of CAOT Publications from *Enabling occupation: An occupational therapy perspective.* 1997).

means of assessing these elements are congruent with the context within which occupational performance will be occurring. For example, assessing someone's ability in the kitchen in the occupational therapy department may not produce outcomes that can be generalized to his or her own kitchen at home; he or she may appear quite confused and slow because he or she cannot find the ingredients, is conscious of being watched, and is in a strange place.

When deciding what to assess and where, it is important to go back to the priority issues as defined in stage 1 and to the theoretical approaches you have chosen to guide you in stage 2.

Stage 4: Identify Strengths and Resources

The purpose of this stage is to gather together all the known strengths and resources that the client brings to the encounter. Similarly, the strengths and resources brought by the therapist and those recognized within the client's support systems warrant being accounted for here.

It is at this stage that occupational therapy service may come to a close if assessment was the purpose of the initial referral. Moving on to stage 5 and beyond will be discussed in Chapter Ten.

MEET JUDY

Judy is a 14-year-old with a diagnosis of spina bifida and hydrocephalus. She uses a manual wheelchair for mobility and is able to maneuver the wheelchair easily. She is independent in all transfers. She is a pleasant, sociable young woman who lives at home with her parents, younger brother, and grandmother. Her father is a long distance truck driver and is seldom home. Her mother receives social assistance, since she has been unemployed for the past 5 years due to health problems, and family finances are poor. The family moved to the area a year ago. The house is split-level—the kitchen, living and dining rooms, bathroom, and three bedrooms are on the main floor; the family room, laundry area, and Judy's bedroom are on the lower level. There is a walk-out, with sliding doors, off the family room to the backyard, which has a swimming pool.

Judy enters and exits her house from the backyard, because there are five steps at the front entrance. Inside the house, there is a stair glide from the lower level to the main floor, but it has not been working for the past 3 months and the family cannot afford to have it repaired. Judy lives on the lower level most of the time, and her mother brings her meals to her. She uses a commode for toileting and the laundry tub for washing. On the weekend, her mother carries her upstairs for a shower.

Judy is in grade 10 in a modified vocational program at a high school that is not in her local community. She is bussed to school every day. Her program involves a modified course load with a special resource class each day to assist her with English and math, which are both difficult subjects for her. Teaching assistants are available for the students in the modified program in each of their classes. This semester, Judy is taking English, math, parenting, and resource classes. The school is physically accessible for Judy and other students in wheelchairs. There is one washroom in an area of the school designated for students receiving resource support, where a teacher coordinates the special services needed by the students in the modified program (e.g., transportation, medications).

➡ What are some of the key concerns/issues you have as an occupational therapist when considering this scenario?

➡ Are there any other health professionals who you feel could be helpful here?

Last year, Judy was seen by an occupational therapist on an outpatient basis at a local rehabilitation center for children and adolescents with physical disabilities. At the beginning of this school year, occupational therapy intervention at school was requested by her resource teacher. School staff were reporting a strong smell of urine most of the time, to the point that staff and students were avoiding getting close to Judy. By the end of the second week of school, her clothes and hair were dirty. They had also noticed that Judy was not bringing a lunch to school most days and bought soda and chips instead from the vending machine. The school staff were getting frustrated and wanted some help in addressing personal hygiene and nutrition issues with Judy. They also wanted an occupational therapy assessment regarding future vocational pursuits as part of transition planning for Judy.

➡ What kinds of assessment tools and approaches would you consider using here in order to identify occupational performance issues?

The occupational therapist conducted an initial assessment of Judy's occupational performance in the school setting, focusing on the issues as identified by Judy, her family, and the school staff.

- Main issues identified by Judy:
  - Being able to use the kitchen to make simple meals and snacks
  - Being able to get out into the community more, like going to the mall with her friends and doing her own shopping

  - ✧ Interested in participating in a work experience program at school
- Main issues identified by her mom were:
  - ✧ Wanted Judy to be more independent at home in self-care
  - ✧ Wanted Judy to do some of her own laundry
- Main issue identified by staff was:
  - ✧ Have Judy pay more attention to good nutritional habits
- Everyone agreed that:
  - ✧ Priority should be given for Judy to gain more control over her bladder and bowel functions

Write up these occupational performance issues, considering the following:

➡ Who is your client?

➡ Who else should you consider?

➡ How should priority be given to these issues?

Selecting Theoretical Approaches

Now, let's consider Judy's situation and what you know about it so far.

➡ What approach (theories, frameworks, models) do you think would be the best to underscore and clarify what you are going to be planning with Judy, her mother, and the staff at her school?

The identification of the occupational performance issues described earlier guided the therapist in selecting the theoretical approaches that would be used throughout the client-centered occupational therapy process. The complex nature of the occupational performance issues called for several different theoretical approaches to be used.

A developmental approach was used to assess performance components and to facilitate discussion of Judy's interests, dreams, and concerns as an adolescent. It was important to be aware of typical adolescent issues; for example, her number-one priority was to do things with her friends. This was her motivation for almost everything she did. Furthermore, she was interested in exploring future vocational directions, which is typical of her age.

A developmental approach also guided the choice of qualitative and quantitative assessment tools. Parts of the Adolescent Role Assessment (Black, 1976) were used to frame interviews to explore Judy's current role performance in areas of school and socialization with family and peers. The occupational therapist also used the Vocational Interest Inventory-Revised (VII-R) (Lunneborg, 1993) to assist Judy in identifying her interests and exploring options for the future. Judy demonstrated the most interest in service areas, as well as arts and entertainment. The occupational area in which she was least interested was technical, science, and organization.

Findings of a comprehensive occupational therapy assessment of performance components and environmental conditions included:

- Few expectations were placed on Judy to be independent at home since Mom did almost everything for her; however, Mom got very angry when things did not go right. She expected Judy to start taking care of herself without special training or support, and Judy felt incompetent and unsure of where and how to start to do more for herself.

- Judy was noted to be friendly and sociable with her peers and chatty with people whom she knows. Lately, she has tended to become tearful when asked about home and personal issues. She said she did not talk with her mom much about such things because her mom tended to get mad at her. She recognized that she would like to work on being able to express her needs to people without getting upset.
- Judy was having some difficulty getting used to the student role in high school. The results of the vocational tests were helpful in identifying future directions.

An environmental approach was also necessary in this case, as there were many issues related to the physical and social environment that were impacting on Judy's occupational performance. Thorough environmental assessments were completed at home and at school:

- Broken stair glide at home prevented Judy from accessing the bathroom and kitchen regularly.
- Bathtub with sliding doors made independent transfers difficult.
- Reliant on mom for transportation; not registered with local disabled transport system.
- Lived in a different community from her friends.
- Mom has fibromyalgia and a sore back, which makes it difficult for her to manage everything.
- Family finances are difficult.
- Has only one T-foam cushion for her wheelchair; despite washing the cover after accidents, the cushion itself has a strong smell of urine.
- Only one washroom at school in a separate "resource" area that had been adapted with a large wheelchair-accessible stall and lowered sink.
- Transportation to and from school was in a special "wheelchair" bus, which limited Judy's participation in social activities.

You will meet Judy again in Chapter Ten, but meanwhile...

Meet Edna

Edna is an 80-year-old African-American woman who lives alone in a one-story home that she owns. There are 10 steps at the front entrance and five at the back. However, the back entrance leads to an alley and the neighborhood is not very safe. Edna has cataracts, high blood pressure, non-insulin-dependent diabetes, and arthritis that affects her knees, hips, and ankles. She is also incontinent. She has a straight cane that she usually uses when ambulating outside her home. Inside her home, she often holds onto furniture to help her move from place to place. Her endurance level is poor, and she is easily fatigued with light to moderate activity.

Edna has a son who is supportive but not involved with the day-to-day care of his mother. Her oldest granddaughter manages Edna's finances and does grocery shopping for her weekly. This granddaughter lives about half an hour away, works full-time, and also has two young children to care for. Edna's sole source of income is her Social Security check of $680 dollars per month. She has assistance from the Division on Aging with personal care and light housekeeping chores. She also has a social worker assigned to coordinate her services.

Recently, Edna has been losing weight, not eating properly, and not taking her medication appropriately. She is on several different kinds of medications for high blood pressure, diabetes, a water pill, some vitamins and iron, and so on. Her granddaughter reports that she will ask the same questions repeatedly and occasionally has word-finding difficulties with common items such as "margarine." She also reports that Edna has been more isolated lately and not able to get out into the community for things like going to church or grocery shopping. She only goes out when going for doctor visits every couple of months. She has not driven for over 13 years and is dependent on someone to take her to her appointments—usually a church member or neighbor to whom she pays a nominal sum for gas. Edna's granddaughter requested occupational therapy services to assess her environment for safety. The granddaughter is afraid that her grandmother's environment is no longer safe and has suggested that she move to a seniors' apartment complex or an assisted living facility. Edna is adamant that she remain in her own home. She states that she would rather die in her house than move to some nursing home where they will "treat you like a dog."

➡ What are some of the possible occupational performance issues that arise when learning about Edna?

- What approach (theories, models, and frameworks) can guide you to approach the issues, which are presented by Edna and her granddaughter, and frame your assessment and potential intervention?

Identify Occupational Performance Components and Environmental Conditions

Now is the point when you can address your concerns about what occupational performance components are problems, and similarly, what elements of Edna's environment can prove to be issues. Remember to identify who the clients are in this situation and from what sources you can glean the most useful information.

- What assessments could you use to find out what you need to know?

Now, let's take a look at what the occupational therapist in this case did use for her assessments and what she found out about Edna.

Using the Canadian Occupational Performance Measure (COPM), Kitchen Task Assessment (KTA), Activity Card Sort (ACS), and observation of functional tasks, as well as observations of the home environment, it was determined that an environmental approach would be taken. These assessments were chosen because they would allow the therapist to understand what the client wants to focus on and provide the opportunity for observation of functional tasks. On the COPM, Edna was able to identify two priority issues:

- Being able to stay in her home, no matter what.
- Being able to get out of the house more often.

The ACS showed that Edna used to go to church, visit sick friends in the hospital, and complete household chores, such as washing dishes, preparing meals, doing laundry, grocery shopping, and managing her finances. Gradually over the past 2 to 3 years, she has given up these things. Currently, her leisure interests include watching television, listening to the radio, and talking on the phone. She will also socialize with friends and relatives if they come to visit. Once or twice a year she will go to her granddaughter's house to visit on special holidays.

On the KTA, Edna had difficulty sequencing the tasks and following the written directions but had good task initiation and was aware of safety at the time of the assessment.

Observations of other functional tasks revealed that Edna was having difficulty being able to get in and out of the bathtub safely. She holds onto the towel rail and has an extremely hard time getting up from the bottom of the tub. She only takes a bath when her personal care attendant is there to assist her. Her kitchen chairs do not have arm rests and when she tries to get up from them she usually pulls up on the table to get from sit to stand. She also has a hard time getting in and out of her bed because there is nothing to hold; therefore, she has chosen to sleep on the couch and uses the arm rest to help her maneuver up and down. There is a rail on one side of the outside steps, but they are very steep and Edna needs physical assistance to manage the stairs. She holds onto the rail but also leans heavily on others for support.

Identifying Strengths and Resources

Are we getting a clear picture of Edna? What you need to do now is identify the strengths that Edna and her family bring to this partnership and then reflect on what you, the therapist, also bring.

- Knowing what you know about Edna, what do you think her strengths are?

Without question, one of Edna's key strengths is her desire to remain in her own home. So often, someone with such a strong commitment to a goal can, by sheer resolution and grit, influence the future. She also exhibits a willingness to make changes to enable her to stay. Her family is concerned and committed to her, particularly one of her granddaughters, and her son is supportive although not frequently present in the immediate environment. Edna has support from the Division on Aging, providing her with home-based services as necessary, and fellow church members and neighbors offer their help in many ways. She lives in a large metropolitan area and has access to a variety of services for seniors and those in the lower income bracket. Although Edna appears to have some mild cognitive deficits, she is able to assist with the direction her care will take.

➡ Knowing what you know about being an occupational therapist in this kind of situation, what strengths do you think you (the therapist) bring to this partnership?

The therapist's strengths are centered around her experience in working with older adults and their families within a community setting. Her special expertise is that of facilitating older adults to optimize the "fit" between their functional abilities and their home and community environments. She also has the knowledge of many resources within the local neighborhood and community, which she can share with Edna and her granddaughter when appropriate and helpful.

In this chapter, we examined in-depth the first four stages of the Occupational Performance Model (Fearing et al., 1997). The following chapter, Chapter Ten, will complete the cycle of the model and address the remaining stages: negotiating targeted outcomes and developing action plans, implementing plans through occupation, evaluating outcomes, and determining any future course of action.

References

Black, M. M. (1976). The adolescent role assessment. *Am J Occup Ther, 30*(2), 73-79.

Canadian Association of Occupational Therapists. (1997). *Enabling occupation: An occupational therapy perspective*. Ottawa, ON: CAOT Publications.

Fearing, G., Law, M., & Clark, J. (1997). An occupational performance process model: Fostering client and therapist alliances. *Canadian Journal of Occupational Therapy, 64*(1), 7-15.

Law, M., Baptiste, S., Carswell, A., McColl, M., Polatajko, H., & Pollock, N. (1998). *Canadian occupational performance measure manual* (3rd ed.). Ottawa, ON: CAOT Publications.

Lunneborg, P. (1993). *The vocational interest inventory, revised (VII-R) manual*. Los Angeles: Western Psychological Services.

Resources

Activity Card Sort (ACS). Baum, C. M. & Edwards, D. F. Edwards, (1993). Available from Dr. Carolyn Baum, Program in Occupational Therapy, Box 8505, Washington University School of Medicine, 4444 Forest Park Blvd., St. Louis, MO 63108.

Kitchen Task Assessment (KTA). Baum, C. M., & Edwards, D. F. (1993). Cognitive performance in senile dementia of the Alzheimer's type: The kitchen task assessment. *Am J Occup Ther, 47*(5), 431-436.

Notes

Chapter Ten

Occupation-Based Practice: Putting It All Together (Part Two)

Mary Law, PhD, OT(c) and Carolyn M. Baum, PhD, OTR/L, FAOTA

Practice Scenario Authors: Kathy Kniepmann, MPH, OTR/L, CHES
Debra Stewart, MSc, OT(c)
Cynthia R. Ballentine, MSOT, OTR/L

In Chapter Nine, we began to describe and apply the Occupational Performance Process Model (Fearing, Law, & Clark, 1997). In Chapter Ten, we continue this process, focusing on the final three steps of the process model and introducing how to document occupation-based practice.

Occupational Performance Process Model

In this chapter, you will learn how to apply this model to defining the outcomes of occupational therapy, planning and carrying out occupation-based interventions, and evaluating occupational performance outcomes after therapy intervention. Additionally, we will offer some examples of how to document treatment and progress that focuses on the occupational goals of the client (Figure 10-1). Let's begin.

Stage 5: Negotiate Targeted Outcomes and Develop Action Plans

In stage 5 of the occupational performance process, the therapist and client (together with the client's family, if involved) develop targeted outcomes. Targeted outcomes are the end results of the therapy intervention as seen by the client and the therapist together. As stated by Fearing and Clark (1998, p. 71) "the therapist and client look ahead and envision a possible client future." Targeted outcomes are stated clearly in terms that the client, therapist, and family can easily understand and in a way that is easily measurable to know if the outcome has been reached. For example, remember Peter's practice scenario in Chapter Seven, whose goal was to return to work as a family physician. Targeted outcomes for him were to return to work 3 days a week within the next 2 months and be able to write medical notes and prescriptions within the time allocated for each patient visit (this time may vary depending on the complexity of the medical issue). You can see that these targeted outcomes reflect Peter's goal of returning to work and it will be easy to set up methods to evaluate if the outcomes have been achieved.

The development of action plans to ensure that the targeted outcome is met is done together by the client and the therapist. The plans focus on resolving the issues related to performance components or environmental conditions that are limiting occupational performance. In Peter's example, his ability to return to work was affected by his endurance and activity levels, so a plan was developed for him to engage in increasing amounts of self-chosen activities and fitness to increase endurance. To improve the targeted outcome related to writing, adaptations for his pens were suggested and a program was designed to increase his upper extremity dexterity, coordination, and endurance. The therapist and Peter visited his workplace to evaluate its accessibility and his office set-up.

Stage 6: Implement Plans Through Occupation

The next step in the process is to implement the action plans through an occupation-based intervention program. Working together so that clients build their problem-solving skills is very important in this stage of intervention. The goal is to enable clients to develop strategies so that they can resolve future occupational performance issues. One of the major challenges for occupational therapists in providing intervention is to ensure that the tasks and activities done during intervention have meaning for the client. This is best achieved through the selection of activities that help improve a performance component and also have meaning to the person. For example, Peter could improve his upper extremity range of motion and strength through a specific exercise regimen or through participation in activities of writing, sports games, gardening, or household remodeling (all interests of his). Choosing the activities route would be more meaningful to him. Plans must be flexible to accommodate changes that may occur along the way (Fearing & Clark, 1998).

Stage 7: Evaluate Occupational Performance Outcomes

The final stage of the occupational performance process focuses on the evaluation of outcomes, identification of any continuing needs, and making future plans. By evaluating outcomes, the therapist finishes a process that begins and ends with occupational performance. Together, the client and therapist evaluate if the occupational performance issues have been resolved. In most situations, this evaluation is best completed using data and information from assessments. For example, for Peter, evaluation data could include a behavioral statement about his return to work, as well as self-assessment of return to work and handwriting using the Canadian Occupational Performance Measure (Law, Baptiste, Carswell, McColl, Polatajko, & Pollock, 1998), and a standardized assessment of writing speed and legibility.

Now is also the time to review the therapy process. Are there any occupational performance issues remaining? If yes, how can they be addressed? What are the client's continuing needs for supporting his or her desired occupations?

Let's examine some practice scenarios and spend time implementing these ideas.

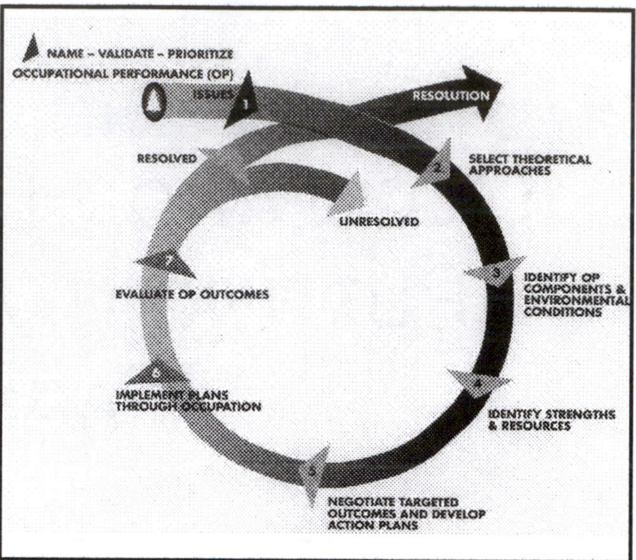

Figure 10-1. Occupational Performance Process Model (adapted from Fearing et al. (1997). *Canadian Journal of Occupational Therapy, 64,* 11, and reproduced with permission of CAOT Publications from *Enabling occupation: An occupational therapy perspective.* 1997).

Meet Judy Again

Negotiate Targeted Outcomes and Develop Action Plans

Judy identified the outcomes that were desired by the client after occupational performance issues that had been identified by her mom and school staff were reviewed. It was important to consider their issues and to inform Judy of other people's expectations and concerns. With this information, Judy was able to set some targeted outcomes. To avoid her feeling overwhelmed, it was agreed to focus on short-term outcomes for the next 3 months (until the Christmas break) and put aside the long-term outcomes for future consideration.

- Judy's short-term outcomes that would be achieved through occupational therapy intervention were:
  - ✧ Judy wanted to find a way to have a shower more often than once per week
  - ✧ Judy wanted to make her own lunch a couple of times a week
  - ✧ Judy wanted to go to a movie with her friends on the weekend
  - ✧ Judy wanted to establish a successful bowel and bladder routine
  - ✧ Judy wanted to manage her own money and shop for basic personal supplies (e.g., shampoo, soap)

  - ✧ Judy wanted to be able to express her needs to other people without becoming upset

➠ Write the targeted outcomes that have been identified so that they are clear, specifically related to an occupational performance issue, and the outcome is measurable.

- Long-term outcomes that Judy identified included:
  - ✧ Doing her own shopping (clothes, personal supplies, food)
  - ✧ Making her own meals in the kitchen at home and eating more nutritiously
  - ✧ Going out into the community with friends independently (i.e., her mom not driving her)
  - ✧ Exploring options for future vocations and participating in a work experience program at school
  - ✧ Doing her own laundry at home

➠ Write the targeted outcomes that have been identified so that they are clear, specifically related to an occupational performance issue, and the outcome is measurable.

Implement Plans Through Occupation

Think about how you, as Judy's therapist, would help her to achieve the targeted outcomes that have been identified through an occupation-based intervention program.

➠ What are some things that you need to do to ensure that the therapy action plans are occupation-based?

➠ Take one or two of the targeted outcomes that have been identified. Outline a specific occupation-based action plan.

✧ Targeted Outcome

✧ Proposed Action Plan

Let's read about what actually happened:

The complex nature of the occupational performance issues facing Judy required the coordinated effort and support of many people. A transition meeting was scheduled with Judy, her mom, school staff, and other professionals who were involved in supporting Judy. The meeting would focus on Judy's goals and making some action plans, including the supports she would need. As Judy was afraid of speaking about herself in front of others, we agreed to work first on her being able to present her needs in a meeting without crying. This became the starting point for Judy to become more in control of her own life—we practiced together first, and then she practiced with a teacher. After a few weeks, she was ready to participate in the team meeting. We presented the short- and long-term goals, and a teaching assistant took notes of an action plan. It was determined at the beginning of the meeting that Judy had the final say in what would be part of the plan. During the meeting, she often looked to other people for support but was able to make some decisions.

At the transition meeting, it was agreed that the home environment was not conducive to Judy developing independence in self-care occupations. In the short-term, the occupational therapist and Judy's mom agreed to investigate funding options to get the stair glide repaired in order for Judy to access the kitchen and bathroom more often. Judy's family was not happy with the home, however, because of the numerous access issues and the finances, and decided that they would have their name placed on a list for subsidized accessible housing in their region. These actions were long-term in nature, and some immediate solutions were needed to attend to Judy's hygiene problems. School staff offered the use of a wheelchair-accessible shower that was in a washroom off of one special education classroom. It had not been used for several years and some equipment, such as a bath bench and hand-held shower hose, would be needed, but otherwise it was readily available. During discussion of Judy's hygiene issues, the school staff suggested that Judy's first class every day could be her resource period, and a personal care program could be set up that she would plan with the occupational therapist and resource teacher. The program would focus on Judy's short-term goals of personal hygiene, bowel and bladder control, making her own lunch, and money management. It would be evaluated after 3 months. The team would then meet to discuss the continuation of the program to work on some of Judy's long-term goals.

The occupational therapist provided consultation to Judy and her teacher to develop and implement her personal care program. Occupational analyses in the area of self-care helped to identify the specific tasks and components involved in showering, other personal hygiene, basic meal-making tasks, and money management. The basic resources needed by Judy were identified and were initially supplied by her mom (e.g., soap, shampoo, and food supplies) until Judy was ready to shop for herself. Special equipment was provided on short-term loan by a vendor who worked closely with the occupational therapist. Transfers were practiced in conjunction with the school physiotherapist to ensure Judy's safety. A referral was made to the nurse at the rehabilitation center to work on a bowel and bladder routine and diet counseling. Once the program began, the occupational therapist met weekly with Judy and the teacher to monitor and suggest changes to ensure success.

To assist Judy in achieving her goal of going out with friends on the weekend, the occupational therapist met with her after school one day to discuss transportation resources and address any concerns her family had. A plan was developed to try one outing, with her mom driving her to the mall to meet her friends. In the meantime, the occupational therapist provided Judy with information on applying for specialized wheelchair transportation in her area.

Context

Occupational therapy intervention was carried out primarily within the school environment, as this was the referral source. The school was physically accessible for Judy and her wheelchair, and the staff was able to make some modifications to ensure her full participation. It was the most amenable to immediate physical modifications to enable Judy to achieve her targeted outcomes. The staff was very receptive to any suggestions made by the occupational therapist.

The home environment impacted on Judy's occupational performance and required consideration by the occupational therapist. It was not wheelchair accessible and finances limited the family's ability to make changes. Judy's ability to be independent in functional tasks was greatly impeded, and this would affect her future development. A special home visit was conducted by the occupational therapist to deal with the barriers to Judy's occupational performance. Funding options were sought to have the stair glide repaired, but on consultation, it was recommended that repair was not the answer, as it was in poor condition—a new stair glide would be needed. As this was not feasible, temporary modifications to the laundry room area, including a new commode and a hand-held attachment for washing in the laundry tub, were made. As Judy would be showering at school during the week, she only needed to use the shower on the main floor on the weekends. A new bath seat was recommended to make transfers more efficient and reduce the amount of assistance her mom needed to provide. Long-term plans to move to a subsidized accessible home were supported with a letter written by the occupational therapist.

Barriers and Feasibility

During the occupational therapy process, numerous barriers had to be overcome to enable Judy to achieve her targeted outcomes. These barriers included elements of the physical, sociocultural, and institutional environments around Judy.

In the physical environment, there were many barriers to independence in self-care and leisure occupations. At school, there was only one wheelchair-accessible washroom. The existence of a wheelchair-accessible shower allowed the personal care program to be developed, but some equipment was needed to allow Judy to shower independently. Several trials of equipment were needed to find the right fit for Judy.

The home environment greatly impeded Judy's occupational performance. The lack of physical access to the main bathroom and kitchen prevented Judy from being able to take care of herself. This lack of access was the main contributor to her personal hygiene and nutrition problems. Both short-term and long-term actions were needed to overcome this major barrier.

Sociocultural barriers also needed to be overcome during the occupational therapy process. First, Judy's own reaction to talking about personal issues, which was crying, had to be overcome for her to be in control of the process. Judy's family also needed some information about spina bifida, bowel and bladder function, and most importantly about the developmental issues facing teenagers to facilitate their acceptance of Judy's needs to be more independent and to be with her friends.

Although school staff had experience with students with special needs, they did not understand why Judy was experiencing personal hygiene problems. The occupational therapist provided information about spina bifida and referred staff to the nurse at the rehabilitation center to learn more about bowel and bladder control. The principal, who ultimately had financial responsibility, needed to understand why some modifications were needed to enable Judy to be independent. Also, staff was initially resistant to the idea of Judy participating in a work experience program, and this required ongoing consultation from the occupational therapist to overcome.

Institutional barriers existed that made it difficult to implement some of the recommendations made by the occupational therapist, particularly in the home environment. Financial supports for equipment and home modifications were limited in number and involved a lengthy process. The lack of accessible housing also meant that Judy's family would be on a long waiting list for affordable adequate housing.

Limited transportation for Judy to get out into the community was a barrier to her participation in leisure activities. She had to rely on her mom to drive her places, and this limited her independence. Judy investigated transportation services for people with physical disabilities with assistance from the occupational therapist. She found it was limited in her community and could not take her to her friends' homes in a different community.

The occupational therapist worked with Judy to overcome these barriers and to build supports in her environments to help her achieve her targeted outcomes.

➡ Think about this action plan. Write down your thoughts about it.

- What aspects of it were particularly effective?

- What aspects were most challenging to the client and therapist?

- What aspects would you do differently and why?

- Are there issues that are similar or different to what you know about occupational therapy practice?

Evaluate Occupational Performance Outcomes

The outcomes of occupational therapy intervention were evaluated after the 3-month, short-term time period. Prior to the team meeting, Judy and the occupational therapist revisited her short-term goals and discussed the process of planning and implementing the personal care program. Judy had maintained a personal journal as part of the program, and her notes were reviewed. Suggestions for change in the process were discussed with the teaching assistant.

Outcomes were evaluated by re-administering the COPM with Judy, her mom, and the teacher. Scores of performance and satisfaction had increased for all three in the areas of self-care and leisure. Productivity (i.e., wanting to find out about working with children in the future) remained unchanged, as this was a long-term goal.

➡ Were Judy's targeted outcomes achieved? Based on your evaluation of the outcomes, was this occupational therapy intervention effective? What are Judy's continuing needs?

➡ How do occupational therapists currently evaluate outcomes after therapy intervention in your practice? Are there any changes you would like to make to the evaluation process? If yes, write your ideas down.

Continuing Needs/Issues

Judy's long-term goals were reviewed at the team meeting, and she felt that they were unchanged. They served as the plan for the remainder of the school year. The occupational therapist continued to provide consultation to Judy and school staff around some of the components of the personal care program (e.g., going out into the community independently and making meals at home). Any adaptive aids needed to increase Judy's independence in making meals were suggested by the occupational therapist. The occupational therapist continued to provide Judy and her family with information about financial supports and specialized community services in their area. As Judy's parents witnessed her improved ability to manage her own money, they agreed to a money management and shopping plan.

The possibility of Judy participating in a work experience program at school next year was discussed, which would provide her with work placement in a day care setting. This would be a first step toward her future productive goal of working with children. School staff agreed to set up a meeting with the co-operative education program staff to start planning. The occupational therapist provided information about spina bifida and hydrocephalus to the program staff, and explained her role in supporting the process through ongoing education and recommendations for modifications to the physical environment. This facilitated everyone's acceptance of Judy applying for this course for the next school year.

In our next practice scenario, we move from a focus on an individual client to a situation where a therapist is working with a community organization. Let's see how the final steps of the process apply when an organization is your client.

Working with the Multiple Sclerosis Society—Negotiate Targeted Outcomes and Develop Action Plans

The initial contact for this project was with the local chapter of the National Multiple Sclerosis Society. Their general goal was to provide resources that would support community functioning of people with multiple sclerosis (MS). They wanted affordable programs and materials, and agreed with these occupational therapists that program planning should be based on goals of the potential participants.

The purpose of this course was to enhance the quality of life for individuals with MS. It would provide opportunities for participants to develop new skills for health promotion and incorporate them into their lifestyles.

Overall goals for participants in the first wellness course were based on phone interviews of the people who expressed interest in the program. Program evaluation results and observation of each session helped the leaders refine the overall course goals and strategies to help participants reach those goals. Before coming to the first session of the 6-week wellness course, participants were each asked to list a goal statement for themselves.

Participants in the wellness course had some shared "goal themes," with variations in their individual goals. Improved ability to cope with fatigue and weakness was a prominent goal for everyone. Maximizing independence in self-care and maintaining productivity was a common general goal, with details varying from person to person. Many of them wanted to garner more social support. They were also seeking techniques to cope with stigma and with the uncertainty of their futures, given the unpredictable symptoms of MS. Stress was a common concern but was prioritized differently by each participant.

Most members talked about their distress with this uncontrolled, unpredictable disease. They had a variety of ways of coping with this lack of control, including guilt, humor, anger, depression, and fear. Most of them hoped to find ways to gain some sense of control, to feel that their lives were their own, and that they could make choices.

➡ Write the targeted outcomes for the group that has been identified so that they are clear, specifically related to an occupational performance issue, and the outcome is measurable.

Implement Plans Through Occupation

As Fearing, Law, and Clark (1997) declare, "the art of occupational therapy includes the ability to create healthy environments where clients can grow and change while remaining firmly grounded within the context of their own lives" (p. 12). The wellness course provided a structure that could let participants address common goals of the group, while also including enough flexibility to deal with the unique contexts and priorities of participants' individual lives. The occupational therapy course leaders facilitated discussions on applying or adapting skills to meet specific needs. They also set the stage for participants to support each other through sharing of ideas, techniques, perspectives, or relevant community resources.

➡ What are some things that you need to consider in this situation to ensure that the therapy action plans are occupation-based?

➡ How is this different when the client is a group of people or an organization that works for them?

➡ Take one or two of the targeted outcomes that have been identified. Outline a specific occupation-based action plan that could be used with a group.

✧ Targeted outcome

✧ Proposed action plan

Let's read about what happened during this group program.

This program was designed to meet group goals in a generic sense, while allowing individual participants the flexibility to focus on their own personal goals. Each person was asked to list at least one personal goal before the course began. At the end of the 6-week course, they were given copies of their own goals and asked to rate how well they reached them.

A key contributor to successful adjustment to living with chronic disease is self-efficacy for self-health management of disease consequences (Clark & Dodge, 1999). Self-efficacy is the belief in one's ability to develop and utilize skills and has been utilized by programs for several different health conditions (Braden, McGlone, & Pennington, 1993; Clark, Becker, Janz, Lorig, Rakowski, & Anderson, 1991; Clark & Dodge, 1999; Dwyer, 1997; Hirano, Laurent & Lorig, 1994; Holman & Lorig, 1997a, 1997b; Lorig & Holman, 1993; Lorig, Mazonson, & Holman, 1993). Lorig's extensive work on self-management courses for people with rheumatoid arthritis, in particular, provided valuable guidance in the development of this course for individuals with MS.

Occupational goal-setting can facilitate skill development and self-efficacy (Gage & Polatajko, 1994). At the end of each session, all participants were asked to set a very specific, measurable goal that they would try to accomplish during the following week. They reported back to the group weekly about that performance and set a new goal. Participants were given several guidelines for goal setting:

- Identify something you want to work on or change.
- Be realistic with your plan (neither overwhelming nor very easy).
- Be specific—what, when, how many, or how much.
- Write the goal in the weekly goal-setting plan.
- Check your goal daily and keep track of what is done.

Individual goals could be based on topics addressed during that session, previous sessions, or other skills related to a person's pursuit of wellness. Many personal goals were related to exercise, stress management, or environmental changes. Examples include getting exercise through adjusted leisure activity, performing class exercise routine several times in the week, taking specific social initiatives, changing the environment of their kitchen or office, and adjusting schedules or routines to accommodate individual needs.

- Intervention content: The class met weekly, 2 hours at a time for 6 weeks. Each session included 30 minutes of guided exercises including:
  - ✧ Flexibility and endurance routines
  - ✧ Exercises that can be done while sitting in a chair
  - ✧ Leisure activities as exercise
  - ✧ Self-monitoring during exercise through use of simple daily exercise diary forms
  - ✧ Methods to adapt routines to suit individual interests, resources, schedules, and changing energy levels
- The course addressed topics germane to occupational performance of group members, including:
  - ✧ Coping with fatigue
  - ✧ Managing productivity, including workplace issues and employee rights under the Americans with Disabilities Act
  - ✧ Coping, stress management, social challenges, psychological issues, and mental health resources
  - ✧ Adapting leisure activities
  - ✧ Cognitive changes and strategies to enhance performance
  - ✧ Communication with health professionals
  - ✧ Getting on the computer superhighway

These topics were explored in a variety of ways, including brief presentations, discussions, and sharing of examples with leaders who facilitate encouragement and problem solving among group members. Emphasis was on application through occupational performance priorities defined by each individual (rather than practice of defined routines) during the week, not just at wellness course sessions. Individual participants supported each other at determining their own individual priorities for wellness and formulating strategies to accomplish their goals.

Context of the Intervention

The wellness course was offered six times over a 3-year period in the St. Louis area before applying for funding to develop a national training program that would develop leaders who could offer more courses. Seventy people took the course in those first 3 years, with an age range from 26 to 66 years, with a mean age of 44. Course participants were primarily females (75%), but included males as well (25%). All of them had at least a high school degree. The average time since diagnosis with MS was 8 years, but some people had been diagnosed within the past year and others had lived with MS for decades.

Use of a health promotion model instead of the medical model guided the course content, educational experiences, and site selection. An empowerment approach involved the clients as active participants in each session, with the course leaders (occupational therapists) facilitating rather than directing the learning process. Participants learned from each other as well as from course leaders. The course was held in community sites rather than at clinics or hospitals. The Program in Occupational Therapy at Washington University provided an ideal location because it also had an adapted apartment/activities of daily living lab where people could discuss and try out assistive technology or home adaptations. A brief introduction to the computer superhighway (Internet) could be held in their technology lab. The wellness course was held several times at that site. Other locations that were used included a college and the meeting room of a community hall.

Several factors were considered as sites were selected. Requirements included:

- Enough open room for a group of 15 to 20 to spread out for exercises.
- Parking located near the building with minimal distance to the classroom, to minimize exertion and fatigue before the course.
- Availability of several accessible parking spaces.
- Fully accessible restrooms nearby.
- Chairs that could be arranged in a large circle for discussions. (It was important to not be restricted by a classroom set-up with chairs in rows facing a lecturer. Face-to-face discussion among participants was essential.)

The course met weekly at the designated location, but the intervention also occurred during the week in each participant's home, workplace, recreation sites, places of worship, and other community settings. The course leaders facilitated discussion of how people could apply the course information and experience to their daily lives. Participants shared information about community resources they found and helped each other with group problem solving. The course was designed to emphasize learning from each other, using supportive "give and take" strategies from social learning theory and empowerment.

"Staffing" included two occupational therapists who designed the course and served as facilitative course leaders during the six sessions. Occupational therapy fieldwork students also helped with the entire course as well as pre- and post-testing. The leaders invited guest speakers (a neurologist and a psychologist) to do brief presentations and discussions.

Barriers and Feasibility

Financial challenges can be barriers to community program development. Occupational therapists who want to develop health promotion and prevention programs in the community need to be very resourceful and persistent at locating funding. In this scenario, the academic occupational therapy program director supported the faculty efforts in developing the new program. Additional costs beyond faculty time (flipcharts, postcards, handouts, name tags) were provided through the occupational therapy program. The initial program was viewed as a pilot community program and evaluation, where students could learn, and faculty and students could explore research questions. After offering the course for free initially, they began charging a nominal registration fee of $25 dollars for each participant. Funding from the local chapter of National Multiple Sclerosis Society (NMSS) supplemented the occupational therapy program support, and the chapter provided increasing amounts of support as they saw outcome data that clarified the positive effects of the course.

At that point, the NMSS chapter was interested in expanding the number of courses, and the faculty in the project could not meet that need. To fund training of additional program leaders, create leader and participant materials, and conduct research of the intervention, the lead occupational therapist on this project investigated grant possibilities. Funding and further support for these needs was secured from the Education & Training Foundation of Paralyzed Veterans of America (ETF/PVA), the NMSS (through a matched grant from the local Gateway Area Chapter, NMSS), and Washington University Program in Occupational Therapy. The course was formally named Gateway to Wellness, A Program for Individuals with Multiple Sclerosis and is completely administered by the NMSS and offered throughout the United States.

Another potential barrier is the attitudes of health professionals who foster dependency on a medical model that emphasizes expert management and cures. This course endorses empowerment of clients, with their active involvement in learning of new self-management skills. Guest speakers need to be carefully selected and coached to give interactive presentations rather than directive lectures.

Publicizing/recruitment can take extra time and effort, but a program done in partnership with a community agency might be able to utilize their resources to accomplish these tasks.

Finding a suitable and attractive community location (see list of criteria on previous page) at a low cost can be difficult. The occupational therapist may need to call a variety of community agencies to find such a site. Community centers or local libraries could be contacted as possibilities.

Staffing could be difficult to find for periodic programs with limited budgets. Occupational therapy fieldwork students helped make this a manageable program, and simultaneously the course provided them with great experience in a new health care paradigm.

Evaluate Occupational Performance Outcomes

Think about the targeted outcomes and action plans that were carried out during this program. Formulate and write down your ideas for evaluating the outcomes of this program.

➠ What information/data would you collect?

➠ How would you collect it?

Let's see what happened.

Multiple measures were used to evaluate program effectiveness. Content and process were examined with subjective and objective measures to identify individual and collective changes. Post-testing was done shortly after course completion, within 10 days of the final session.

Program evaluations were very positive. Many participants applauded the opportunity to share information and ideas with others who knew what it was like to live with MS. They learned by doing—on their own as well as with others and from others. They felt that the goal setting at the end of each session helped them to gain a sense of accomplishment and control. The high attendance and low dropout rates were also testimony to the satisfaction and strong investment in this program. By the end of the course, the majority of participants reached the personal goals that they set initially.

Participants had the opportunity to give each other encouragement and feedback about their goals. They also collaborated at problem solving and adjusting perspectives, helping each other structure occupational roles and behaviors that were personally meaningful for their own wellness. Some participants found it difficult to change their expectations and behavior patterns, and tended to view such adjustment as failure. At times, others in the group could help them reframe their perspectives. For instance, one person reported back that she failed at her goal of exercising three times in the week for at least 20 minutes. She explained that she needed to do housecleaning for a family event and had to walk the dog when her husband worked late. Other participants suggested that although she did not do the exercise routine that she planned, she certainly did physical exercise in the performance of these responsibilities. People with MS were very receptive to giving and receiving information from others with MS who shared similar occupational performance issues. For people who live in the community without the label of patient/client, this was more powerful input than individual therapy from an expert clinician.

Stories from participants demonstrated many important contributions that this course made to the quality of their lives in a variety of ways. One woman said that the only experience that was more meaningful and valuable in her whole life than this wellness course was having her baby. Several commented about how valuable it was to meet others with MS and learn how they were coping with it. Many participants explained specific ways they changed their lifestyles as a result of the knowledge and especially the skills they acquired from this course. Decreased fatigue with improved strength and balance were commonly experienced with participation in the exercise program. One woman was very pleased by her increased fitness as well as what she learned about adaptive equipment. She said that it made a marvelous difference in her independence—particularly that she was able to get in and out of the bathtub when no one was home. A banker said that he was able to work full days productively again after beginning an exercise routine and applying work simplification/energy conservation principles. Another woman reported back a year later that she has been exercising every day and feeling better than ever.

Wellness course participants, by the end of the course, showed positive trends in the Assessment of Motor and Process Skills (AMPS) and the Fatigue Scale, as well as the Self-Efficacy Scale for self-management of consequences of MS. As part of the Self-Efficacy Scale after the course, participants reported more confidence in ability to:

- Manage fatigue.
- Continue most daily activities.
- Perform specific self-care and home management tasks.
- Join a new social group.
- Regulate activities in order to be active without aggravating MS symptoms.
- Manage MS symptoms so they could do the things they enjoy.

Data from the Health Status Survey, SF-36, done pre- and immediate post-course, did not reveal significant improvement. Possibly, the measure was not sensitive to identifying changes from the intervention, or possibly the post-test should be given after a longer time period after completion of the wellness course. The Beck Depression Inventory (Beck & Beamesderfer, 1974) showed that no participants were within the clinical depression range. The evaluation battery has been changed further as the Gateway to Wellness program was evaluated on a national basis.

Continuing Issues/Needs

This section will be examined in terms of the continuing issues/needs of the community defined first as the specific program participants, then in terms of the issues and needs of the population that has MS locally, then extended to include the region and the nation.

Issues and Needs of Program Participant:

This wellness course was promoted as a short-term self-management course to build skills and help people learn about community resources. For most participants, the 6-week course was an adequate length to catalyze significant changes. They reported that it gave them a jump-start at building on their own resources for a healthier lifestyle. The wellness course incorporated Baum and Law's (1997) changing health system paradigm by emphasizing a partnership for health management and prevention of disability, emphasizing personal responsibility and choice by clients.

The course was built on an empowerment approach. People with MS were encourage to take charge of their lives by defining their own occupational performance priorities, then develop skills or change their environments to implement those priorities. Although the participants gained many benefits during the 6-week course, many wished that the course lasted longer. They valued the camaraderie and the support enormously. Consequently, many of them kept in touch with varying degrees of regularity. Some began utilizing other resources from the MS society: the aquatics program, support groups, volunteering, participation in education events, and more. They also shared information about environmental accessibility and community resources that could meet their needs and occupational priorities.

Advocacy/self-advocacy was an issue that was difficult for some participants, and others provided guidance or support. Finding affordable or accessible resources was also a concern. Again, some participants were able to help on this.

Changes to Issues and Needs of Leaders

Overall, approximately 250,000 to 350,000 people in the United States have MS (NMSS, ...). The Gateway to Wellness, A Course for Individuals with Multiple Sclerosis is a valuable program for health promotion and self-management of MS. Several continuing needs and issues require attention, such as:

- Training of more course leaders and co-leaders to expand the number of courses throughout the country. Currently, there are plans to offer a Train the Trainer course along with the next Leader Training Program. This would allow wider dissemination of the model.
- Support for leaders and co-leaders as they offer courses with their local chapters of NMSS. E-mail, phone consultation, and mailings provide a means of discussing concerns or exploring strategies to handle challenges. Additional mechanisms may be developed.
- Efficacy has been measured and is being more carefully assessed with comparison to a control group. Findings will clarify outcomes for further refinement of the course.

➡ Think about opportunities for you to develop group programs. List some ideas.

✧ What process will you use to begin to develop these opportunities?

Let's meet Edna again, who is at the center of our final practice scenario.

Negotiate Targeted Outcomes and Develop Action Plans

As you recall, Edna is an 80-year-old African-American woman who lives alone in a one-story home that she owns. There are 10 steps at the front entrance and five at the back entrance. However, the back entrance leads to an alley and the neighborhood is not very safe. She has cataracts, high blood pressure, non-insulin-dependent diabetes, and arthritis that affects her knees, hips, and ankles. She is also incontinent. She has a straight cane that she usually uses when ambulating outside of her home. Inside her home she often holds onto furniture to help her move from place to place. Her endurance level is poor, as she is easily fatigued with light to moderate activity.

After the initial assessment and interview with Edna and her granddaughter, the results were discussed. Edna and her granddaughter identified the issues that were of concern to them, and the therapist identified potential problem areas. In collaboration with Edna, her granddaughter, and the therapist, the following goals were established. Edna's primary goal was to stay in her home and not have go to a nursing home. Another goal was to be able to access her community more and not be confined to her house so much (e.g., go to church more often). A final goal was to be as safe as possible in her home so that her family would not have to worry about her being alone in her house.

➠ Take the targeted outcomes that have been identified and outline a specific occupation-based action plan.

- ✧ Targeted outcome

- ✧ Proposed action plan

Implement Plans Through Occupation

Let's see what was done.

Modifications to Environment

Recommendations for environmental adaptations were as follows:

- Remove phone cord from walkway and get a cordless phone so that the need for a long cord is diminished.
- Have Edna use a large 1-week pill box and have her granddaughter set up her medicines weekly.
- Take up plastic runners and throw rugs to remove fall hazards.
- Increase lighting and bulb wattage as well as placing more direct lighting around the living area.
- Use a bed bar to assist the client with getting in/out of bed. Also provide education to Edna and her granddaughter on the best bed mobility strategies for Edna.
- Install another rail at the steps to the front entrance of the home.
- Install a transfer tub bench and hand-held shower in the bathroom. Also provide training on using equipment to Edna and her personal care aide.
- Have Edna get at least one chair with arms to assist with sitting and standing.
- Suggest that Edna not use a swivel rocking chair. Recommend a recliner, since she currently spends the greater portion of the day in the rocker. A recliner is more comfortable to sit in than a hard straight-back chair with arm rests and is more stationary. If the chair is more stationary, it may prevent falls.
- Suggest Edna and her granddaughter look at reducing the congestion and clutter by removing rarely used furniture and rearranging furniture to allow a wider walkway.
- Provide Edna and her granddaughter with a list of community resources to assist with modifications.
- Provide Edna's granddaughter with information about cognitive loss in older adults and ways to make Edna's environment more supportive.
- Provide her granddaughter with resources on where to purchase adaptive equipment and possible funding sources.

Strategies for Increased Community Access

- Work with her granddaughter to set up a system for family members, church members, and neighbors to help get Edna to church twice a month initially and more often over time.

- Recommend Edna and granddaughter discuss making arrangements for Edna to go to grocery store with her granddaughter once a month. Also recommend that Edna use a wheelchair for these outings because of decreased endurance.
- Provide Edna and her granddaughter with lists of senior centers close to her that have programming during the day. Also discuss transportation alternatives.

Strategies for Home Safety

- Provide Edna and her granddaughter with information on Life-line and how this system works.
- Recommend Edna become part of safe neighbor program at her church, where someone from her church would be called everyday to check on her and she could call others to check on them.
- Recommend physical therapy to assess gait and the need for more supportive assistive devices for ambulation.

Context

The intervention generally occurred in Edna's home. The therapist assessed Edna's ability to function in her home and ways that the environment was not supporting her. Another aspect of this was also the social context. This involved Edna's granddaughter, church members, and neighbors. Edna's granddaughter was provided with the resources available in the community, and involvement of the members of Edna's support system were incorporated into her intervention plan. The plan could not be implemented without their willingness to participate.

Evaluate Occupational Performance Outcomes

The outcomes of the intervention were that, after making some of the suggested changes, Edna and her granddaughter felt more comfortable with Edna's safety in the home. At 6 months post-intervention, Edna and her granddaughter had removed the throw rugs and plastic runners, shortened the phone cord so that it did not cross the pathway, and added more lighting. The Arthritis Foundation was contacted and was able to provide Edna with a bath bench. They also reported slowly working on getting rid of some of the unused furniture and clothing in Edna's home. Edna is reluctant to get rid of things.

Edna's access to her community has also increased. Edna's granddaughter talked with Senior Home Security and was able to have another rail installed at the front steps free of charge. She generally makes it to church once or twice a month when the weather permits and goes out monthly with her granddaughter to do grocery shopping. She reports that she feels like she is able to do more and does not get tired as fast. She has not yet contacted any senior center programs, but her granddaughter reports that she has been asking about visiting one or two in the near future. She is now a member of the safe neighbor program at her church and enjoys talking to other church members daily. They were not able to afford the Life-line program, the bed bar, or recliner at this time.

Continuing Issues/Needs

Although some environmental changes have occurred, further changes may be beneficial to Edna. She wants to get a bed bar at some point so that she can sleep in her bed again. She is also interested in learning to use her microwave to cook meals because she is getting nervous about using her stove. She has burnt a couple of pots recently, because she forgot and left the stove on too long.

Edna may need a cognitive work-up by her physician to check for further cognitive changes.

Barriers and Feasibility

One barrier that needed to be overcome was Edna's finances. She has a very limited income for her current needs. Another barrier was the poor "fit" she had with her environment. It was not very supportive for her, given her abilities and limitations. Other barriers were her limited family support, decreased cognitive abilities, and her insecurity moving around outside of her home. However, with prioritizing the main issues and making inexpensive modifications, Edna was able to overcome some of her barriers and achieve her primary goal of staying in her home.

We hope that you have developed an understanding of how to apply the Occupational Performance Process Model to planning and implementing occupational therapy programs.

Stage 8: Documenting Occupation-Based Practice

Occupational therapists using an occupation-based approach use activities and tasks familiar to the person to support learning new skills that overcome the limitations imposed by impairments. An occupation-based approach supports the enabling process (Brandt & Pope, 1997) by providing functional restoration and environmental modifications. The occupational therapist must document how the client-centered plan will address the impairment and lead to a functional outcome. The following elements are basic to good documentation practices, can support both an occupation-based approach and meet the expectations of client-centered practice (Law, Baptiste, & Mills, 1995), and meet the criteria for thirdparty documentation. Additionally, such documentation makes the unique contribution of occupational therapy explicit.

Key Elements of the Occupational Therapy Plan

1. Indicate that the client was referred for occupational therapy evaluation and treatment.
2. Summarize the medical conditions and dates of significant medical events.
3. Describe the person and give a brief social and occupational history.
4. Identify precautions to be considered in treatment.
5. Summarize what the client believes has happened to him or her.
6. Report the client's goals (e.g., using the COPM). For each goal, give the performance and satisfaction score.
7. Evaluation results (report findings of each assessment or structured observation).
8. Summarize the client's behavior during the evaluation and treatment planning process.
9. Summarize the person, environment, and activity capabilities.
10. Summarize the person, environment, and activity problems.
11. State the goals agreed upon by the client and practitioner. (Integrate client goals with problems that need attention and state in functional and measurable terms.)
12. Describe the plan for treatment.

Key Elements of the Progress Note

1. Subjective information: State how the client perceives the plan and report what he or she finds helpful or problematic.
2. Report on the status of each previous goal.
3. Revisit the COPM to see if the client has additional issues that need to be addressed.
4. Jointly establish functional and measurable goals to be accomplished in the next phase of treatment.
5. Describe the plan that will be used to address the goals.

Key Elements of the Discharge Note

1. Subjective Information: Report the client's assessment of the treatment experience.
2. Report the follow-up on the COPM.
3. Report the status of goals (use functional and measurable terms).
4. Indicate the planning for community support and follow-up.

The following provides some examples of how to document the problem and goal:

- Problem
  - ✧ Decreased range of motion
- Client goal
  - ✧ Be able to wash face, comb hair, work in kitchen, braid her child's hair, and hang clothes on the line
- Documented goal
  - ✧ In 2 weeks, the client will demonstrate active range of motion in shoulder flexion/abduction above 100 degrees while completing home management tasks, such as putting groceries in the cupboard or hanging laundry on the line
- Documentation: Mrs. Jones continues to show improvement in her shoulder motion, achieving 85 degrees of shoulder flexion/abduction; however, she continues to be limited in her grooming and homemaking tasks. She is learning to manage pain as we grade the tasks that are presented to increase her tolerance for pain, endurance for tasks, and movement. We expect continued improvement over the next two to three visits. She is complying with progressive exercise and activity recommendations in her home program.

➡ How is this note different from the note you would write now?

- Problem
  - ✧ Difficulty initiating a task
- Client goal
  - ✧ To be able to do things around the house so that his daughter's family will allow him to continue to live in their home
- Documented goals
  - ✧ Mr. Smith will be able to take his pills using external cues and an alarm on his watch
  - ✧ He will be able to use posted signs in the bathroom to initiate his grooming tasks

    - ✧ Mr. Smith and his daughter will set up a "station" where his cards to play solitaire, the daily paper, and the labeled TV remote are located so that he will have items at the point of use
- Documentation: Mr. Smith requires external cues to begin to do activities that he was able to complete before his transient ischemic attack. The focal lesion has interfered with his ability to initiate tasks and limits his independent function. His initial goals are simple, as he does not want to be a burden on his daughter, who must get the children ready for school and leave for work by 7:45 a.m. He has made progress, as he now recognizes that he has a problem initiating tasks and is willing to learn to use external stimuli as reminders.
- Plan: In order to gain independence in initiation, it will be necessary for Mr. Smith to use environmental strategies. Over the next five visits, Mr. Smith will practice using external cues to initiate tasks that are important to his basic self-care function and daily activities. The family will help by learning the cues to support Mr. Smith in achieving his goals.

➠ How is this note different from the note you would write now?

- Problem
    - ✧ Poor contrast sensitivity, making it difficult to recognize edges of objects and seeing objects on the same color surfaces; at risk for falls
- Client goal
    - ✧ Go to the basement to do laundry. Prepare scrapbooks from old pictures for her grandchildren, organize her recipes for a family cookbook, choose her clothes so she is not embarrassed by going out of the house with, for example, one navy and one black shoe
- Documented goals
    - ✧ The client will use increased task lighting for home management, grooming, and dressing tasks, and will use the stairs only with lights on at the top and bottom of the steps
    - ✧ The family will install a clothes chute so that she will not need to carry a basket on the steps
    - ✧ Her clothes will be labeled so she can recognize the difference in colors

Now it is your turn. Write a progress note for the above scenario.

➠ Documentation

References

Baum, C., & Law, M. (1997). Occupational therapy practice: Focusing on occupational performance. *Am J Occup Ther, 51*(4), 277-288.

Beck, A. T., & Beamesderfer, A. (1974). Assessment of depression: The depression inventory. *Mod Probl Pharmacopsychiatry, 7*, 151-169.

Braden, C. J., McGlone, K., & Pennington, F. (1993). Specific psycho-social and behavioral outcomes from the Systemic Lupus Erythematosus Self-Help course. *Health Educ Q, 20*(1), 29-41.

Brandt, E. Jr., & Pope, A. (1997). *Enabling America: Assessing the role of rehabilitation science and engineering*. Washington, DC: National Academy Press.

Canadian Association of Occupational Therapists. (1997). *Enabling occupation: An occupational therapy perspective*. Ottawa, ON: CAOT Publications ACE.

Clark, N. M., Becker, M. H., Janz, N. K., Lorig, K., Rakowski, W., & Anderson, L. (1991). Self-management of chronic disease by older adults. *Journal of Aging and Health*, 3(1), 3-27.

Clark, N. M., & Dodge, J. A. (1999). Exploring self-efficacy as a predictor of disease management. *Health Education & Behavior*, 26(1), 72-89.

Dwyer, K. A. (1997). Psychosocial factors and health status in women with rheumatoid arthritis: Predictive models. *Am J of Prev Med, 13*(1), 66-72.

Fearing, G., & Clark, J. (1998). The client-centered occupational therapy process. In: M. Law (Ed.), *Client centered occupational therapy*. Thorofare, NJ: SLACK Incorporated.

Fearing, G., Law, M., & Clark, J. (1997). An occupational performance process model: Fostering client and therapist alliances. *Canadian Journal of Occupational Therapy, 64*(1), 7-15.

Gage, M., & Polatajko, H. (1994). Enhancing occupational performance through an understanding of perceived self-efficacy. *Am J of Occup Ther, 48*(5), 452-461.

Hirano, P. C., Laurent, D. D., & Lorig, K. (1994). Arthritis patient education studies, 1987-1991: A review of the literature. *Patient Education and Counselling, 24*(1), 9-54.

Holman, H. R., & Lorig, K. R. (1997a). Overcoming barriers to successful aging: Self-management of osteoarthritis. *West J Med, 167*(4), 265-268.

Holman, H. R., & Lorig, K. R. (1997b). Patient education: Essential to good health care for patients with chronic arthritis. *Arthritis Rheum, 40*(8), 1371-1373.

Law, M., Baptiste, S., Carswell, A., McColl, M., Polatajko, H., & Pollock, N. (1998). *Canadian Occupational Performance Measure* (3rd ed.). Ottawa, ON: CAOT Publications ACE.

Law, M., Baptiste, S., & Mills, J. (1995). Client-centered practice: What does it mean and does it make a difference? *Canadian Journal of Occupational Therapy*, 62, 250-257.

Lorig, K. (1993). Self-management of chronic illness: A model for the future. *Generations, 17*(3), 11-14.

Lorig, K., & Holman, H. (1993). Arthritis self-management studies: A twelve-year review. *Health Educ Q, 20*(1), 17-28.

Lorig, K. R., Mazonson, P. D., & Holman, H. R. (1993). Evidence suggesting that health education for self-management in patients with chronic arthritis has sustained health benefits while reducing health care costs. *Arthritis Rheum, 36*(4), 439-446.

National Multiple Sclerosis Society. (2001). Sourcebook-Epidemiology. Retrieved from http://www.nationalmssociety.org/Sourcebook-Epidemiology.asp.

Notes

Notes

Section Five

EVALUATING

Although this section contains only one chapter, it is in many ways the culmination of a rich process of reflection and application in which you, the reader, have engaged. At this time in the evolution of the profession of occupational therapy, the critical importance of individual practitioners taking responsibility for their continuing competence cannot be minimized. We have striven for that niche of professional autonomy that is now within our grasp, and we have the tools and knowledge with which to make a noticeable impact on emerging health care systems. However, part of that responsibility and privilege—and it is a privilege—is manifested in our individual abilities to pursue a clearly articulated self-development and self-assessment path. Therefore, Chapter Eleven has been designed to facilitate practice of this essential skill.

Chapter Eleven

A Self-Assessment of Your Learning

Sue Baptiste, MHSc, OT(c) and Mary Law, PhD, OT(c)

You have reached the final stage in your self-paced learning journey. Throughout the past 10 chapters, you explored occupational therapy practice and examined the ways in which we can ensure that practice is one that is client-centered and based in occupational performance. Now is the time to reflect back on your learning, assess the meaning and implications of the self-study for your practice, and evaluate your strengths and future learning needs.

Applying the Occupational Performance Process Model

In this section, you will use the format of the Occupational Performance Process Model (Fearing, Law, & Clark, 1997) that you learned about in Chapters Nine and Ten, and apply it to a practice scenario of your own choice. Think about a client, group, or organization that you have met, worked with, or with whom you are just beginning to work. Using the guided questions that follow, think about the occupational therapy process that you could use and apply it to the scenario that you have identified.

Stage 1: Name, Validate, and Prioritize Occupational Performance Issues

➡ Describe your scenario.

➡ What are some of the key concerns you have when considering this scenario?

- Are there any other health professionals who you feel could be helpful here?

- How will you gather information about the occupational performance issues in this situation?

- Who is your client?

- What are the occupational performance issues?

- How should priority be given to these issues?

Stage 2: Select Theoretical Approach(es)

Now, consider your client's situation: What you know so far is...

- What approaches (theories, frameworks, models) do you think would be the best to underscore and clarify what you are going to be planning with this client?

- How will this approach(es) influence further assessment and intervention?

Stage 3: Identify Occupational Performance Components and Environmental Conditions

Think about the performance components and/or environmental conditions that are influencing occupational performance for this client.

Table 11-1 Left Side—Right Side Diagram

Occupational Performance Issues	*Performance Components/Environmental Conditions*
•	•
•	•
•	•

➠ What further assessment is needed?

➠ What assessments could you use to find out performance components and environmental conditions in this practice scenario?

Construct a left side—right side diagram (Fearing, 1993) to illustrate the possible relationship between occupational performance issues (OPIs) and performance components and/or environmental conditions (Table 11-1).

Stage 4: Identify Strengths and Resources

Think about your client and yourself as a therapist. What strengths and resources do each of you bring to this therapy encounter? What resources are available in the community?

➠ Knowing what you know about this client, what do you think his or her strengths and resources are?

➠ Knowing what you know about being an occupational therapist in this kind of situation, what strengths do you think you (the therapist) bring to this partnership?

➠ What community resources could help in this situation?

Stage 5: Negotiate Targeted Outcomes and Develop Action Plans

Think about the targeted outcomes in your scenario. Remember to write them so that they are clear and measurable.

- Write the targeted outcomes that have been identified so that they are clear, specifically related to an occupational performance issue, and the outcome is measurable.

Think about the action plan that will help this client to achieve these targeted outcomes through an occupation-based intervention.

- Take the targeted outcomes that have been identified. Outline a specific occupation-based action plan.
  - ✧ Targeted outcome
  - ✧ Proposed action plan

Stage 6: Implement Plans Through Occupation

Think about how you, as the therapist, would ensure that intervention is effective and occupation-based.

- What are some things that you need to do to ensure that the therapy action plans are occupation-based?

Use this next space to keep a record of the intervention plan. What worked well? What changes did you and the client make as intervention progressed?

- Reflect on your action plan. Write down your thoughts about it—what aspects of it might work well? What aspects will be most challenging to the client and therapist?

Stage 7: Evaluate Occupational Performance Outcomes

- Plan and write down how outcomes will be measured in this situation.

Know-Can-Do: A Creative Approach to Self-Assessment

One of the key elements of any self-directed process is to evaluate oneself against a set of identified rules, guidelines, or standards that will provide an idea of what has been learned and what should be pursued further. Also, action plans should be made in order to proceed with a defined learning plan, complete with time lines, potential resources, and means of determining that something has been achieved. And so, we will explore a creative model for facilitating such a process, known as "know-can-do" (Norman, 1991).

An essential responsibility of any profession is to establish standards of competence to ensure the general public, members of the professions, and employers that all licensed or certified professionals who provide services to the public are competent (Baum & Gray, 1988; Norman, 1991). Clinical competence in the health disciplines is generally accepted as a combination of knowledge, skills, professional judgment, and behavior (Edwards & Baptiste, 1987).

Norman (1991) has outlined a simple "know-can-do" hierarchical model that is helpful in understanding the complex construct of clinical competence. In this model, knowledge is at the bottom of the hierarchy and is traditionally measured using written tests. Although knowledge is essential for the upper skill and performance levels, there is no guarantee that because someone "knows" how to do something that he or she is actually able to perform the defined skill or demonstrate the particular behavior. The middle "can" level of the hierarchy is used to describe specific technical and professional skills and is usually measured using direct observation methods in real or simulated client encounters. The "do" level is the highest level since it reflects day-to-day practice behavior or performance outside of a test situation; chart audits, client satisfaction surveys, individual learning contracts, and supervisor ratings are often used to measure competence at this level. This is where this model comes into the whole process of which you have been a part while you have gone through this workbook.

In this next section, you will find a set of "I" statements, which you will notice are based upon the process inherent within this study module. These statements are intended to help you reflect on your level of comfort in your understanding of the ideas presented here. The reflective process in which you are going to be engaged is described as follows:

- Read the item carefully and ask yourself, "How comfortable am I with my own knowledge and understanding of this item?"
- Think about what it is upon which you are basing your sense of comfort or discomfort and translate that into your current level by rating yourself on the 7-point scale referred to as the "know-can-do" scale. Basically, you are reflecting on whether you know something, believe that you can institute this change, or already do this in your practice.
- Once you have rated your current level, you need to think about whether you need to or want to be performing at a higher level—this is conveyed in the rating you give yourself on your desired level using the same scale. After you have determined your current and desired levels, you need to consider how you could demonstrate that you are functioning at this level. A number of these indicators may be part of your own self-assessment dossier or portfolio that you choose to develop as an ongoing resource for your continued learning.
- Finally, if you have noted a difference between your current and desired level, then a learning need or follow-up action is probably a sound idea. You need to reflect what you plan to do on your self-learning contract (Table 11-2).

Items for Self-Assessment

Know: 1
Can: 2, 3
Do: 4, 5, 6, 7

- I am aware of trends within society and the occupational therapy profession which are impacting my practice.

  Current level: (circle) 1 2 3 4 5 6 7
  Desired level: (circle) 1 2 3 4 5 6 7

- I can identify the beliefs and values underlying my practice.

  Current level: (circle) 1 2 3 4 5 6 7
  Desired level: (circle) 1 2 3 4 5 6 7

- I understand what client-centered practice looks like.

  Current level: (circle) 1 2 3 4 5 6 7
  Desired level: (circle) 1 2 3 4 5 6 7

- I understand the difference between occupation and task or activity.

  Current level: (circle) 1 2 3 4 5 6 7
  Desired level: (circle) 1 2 3 4 5 6 7

- I am comfortable in using the term "occupation" in my everyday practice.

  Current level: (circle) 1 2 3 4 5 6 7
  Desired level: (circle) 1 2 3 4 5 6 7

Table 11-2 Self-Learning Contract

- Item:
  - ✧ Needs/barriers:
  - ✧ Strategies:
  - ✧ Plan:
- Item:
  - ✧ Needs/barriers:
  - ✧ Strategies:
  - ✧ Plan:
- Item:
  - ✧ Needs/barriers:
  - ✧ Strategies:
  - ✧ Plan:
- Item:
  - ✧ Needs/barriers:
  - ✧ Strategies:
  - ✧ Plan:
- Item:
  - ✧ Needs/barriers:
  - ✧ Strategies:
  - ✧ Plan:

- I understand the elements inherent in a move from a medical/diagnostic practice model to one based on occupational performance.
  Current level: (circle) 1 2 3 4 5 6 7
  Desired level: (circle) 1 2 3 4 5 6 7
- I understand how to reframe my assessments in a client-centered way.
  Current level: (circle) 1 2 3 4 5 6 7
  Desired level: (circle) 1 2 3 4 5 6 7
- I understand the term "targeted outcomes."
  Current level: (circle) 1 2 3 4 5 6 7
  Desired level: (circle) 1 2 3 4 5 6 7

- I can identify the resources I will need to continue along this learning path.

  Current level: (circle) 1 2 3 4 5 6 7
  Desired level: (circle) 1 2 3 4 5 6 7

Let's finish by taking the items for which you have identified a learning need and plan your action(s) to meet that need (see Table 11-2).

You have completed this workbook. We hope that you have found it both challenging and useful. We welcome your feedback.

References

Baum, C. M., & Gray, M. S. (1988). Certification: Serving the public interest. *Am J Occup Ther, 42*, 77-79.

Edwards, M., & Baptiste, S. (1987). The occupational therapist as a clinical teacher. *Canadian Journal of Occupational Therapy, 54*, 249-255.

Fearing, V. G. (1993). Occupational therapists chart a course through the health record. *Canadian Journal of Occupational Therapy*, 60, 232-240.

Fearing, G., Law, M., & Clark, J. (1997). An occupational performance process model: Fostering client and therapist alliances. *Canadian Journal of Occupational Therapy*, 64(1), 7-15.

Norman, G. R. (1991). Can an examination predict competence? The role of recertification in maintenance of competence. *Annals of the Royal College of Physicians and Surgeons of Canada, 24*, 121-124.

Notes

Index